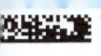

AF173497

DT.NATASHA MOHAN'S

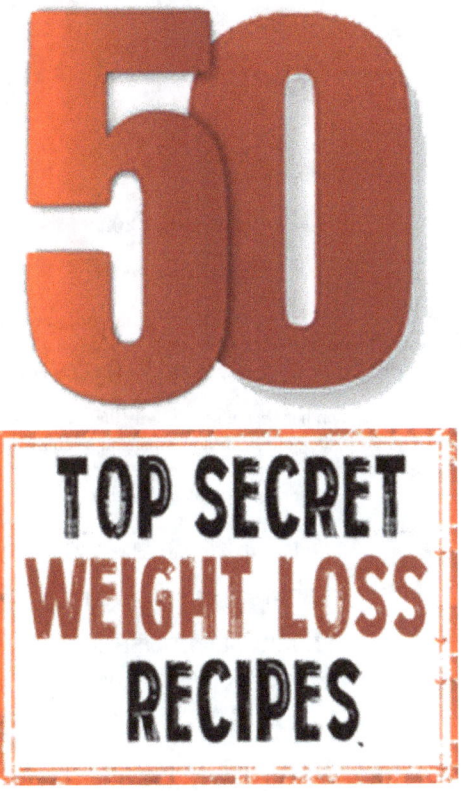

TOP SECRET WEIGHT LOSS RECIPES

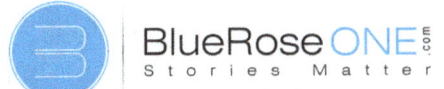

BlueRose ONE_{.co}
Stories Matter

First Published in November 2022

ISBN: 978-93-5704-216-1

BLUEROSE PUBLISHERS
www.BlueRoseONE.com
info@bluerosepublishers.com
+91 8882 898 898

Cover Design:
Natasha Mohan

Typographic Design:
Namrata Saini

Distributed by: BlueRose, Amazon, Flipkart

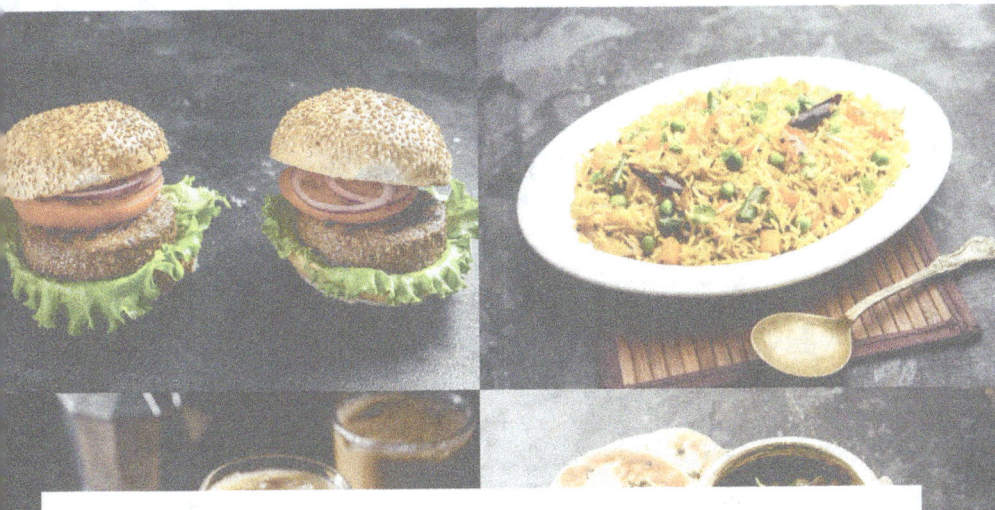

Acknowledgement

I would like to thank and acknowledge my subscribers, who have supported me immensely throughout this journey and motivated me to write this book. I also want to acknowledge my family for supporting me with this book and having faith in me. And finally, I want to acknowledge the editor and publisher of this book, who helped me finalise my book.

It took me so much time to perfect these recipes. If you are new to this journey, I encourage you to closely follow the recipes and you'll get great results. Nothing gives me more pleasure than sharing these healthy recipes and motivating you all to lead a healthy life.

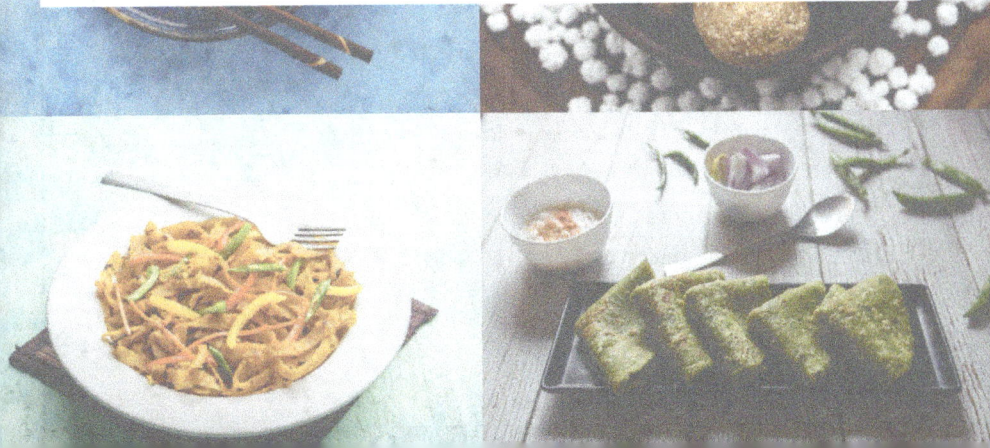

Contents

INTRODUCTION

BEVERAGES

SNACKS

BREAKFAST

LUNCH

Cucumber Coconut Salad	59
Dahi Bhalla	61
Fried Rice	63
Goli Idli	65
Kulchey Choley	66
Lemon Rice	69
Paneer Roll	71
Quinoa Chickpea Salad	73
Spinach & Sprouts Uttapam	75
Stuffed Aloo Parantha	76
Stuffed Parantha	78
Tawa Pulao	80

DINNER

Burger	84
Chilly Paneer	87
Dahi Ke Kebab	89
Oats & Dal Dosa	91
Paneer Makhani	92
Pearl Millet Salad	95
Sama Rice Salad	97
Veg Biryani	98

NON-VEG SPECIALS

Chicken Curry	102
Chicken Tikka	105
Mexican Chicken Wrap	106
Tandoori Fish	108

DESERTS

Carrot Laddoo	113
Dates & Almond Laddoo	115
Kheer	117

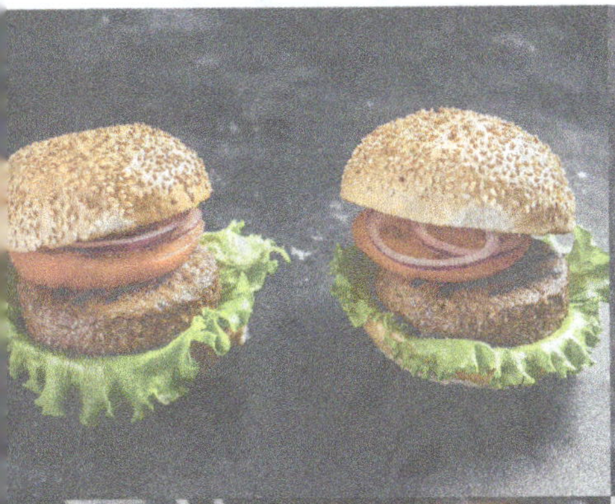

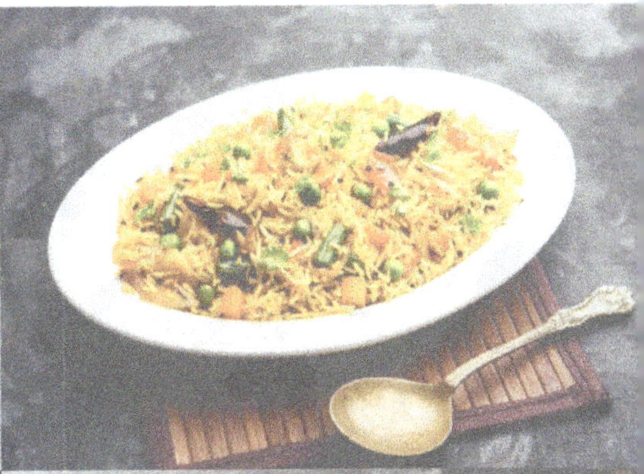

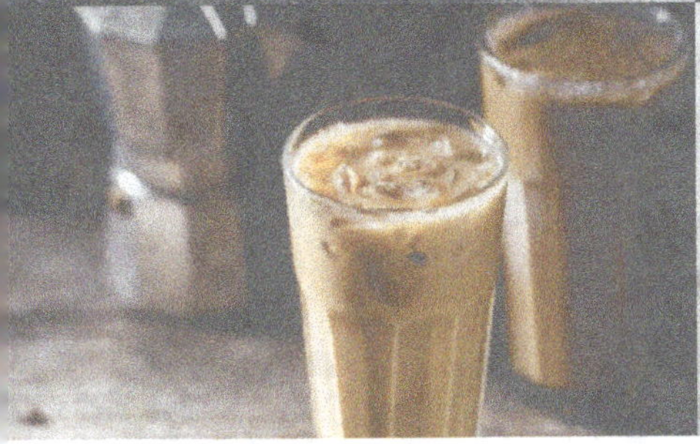

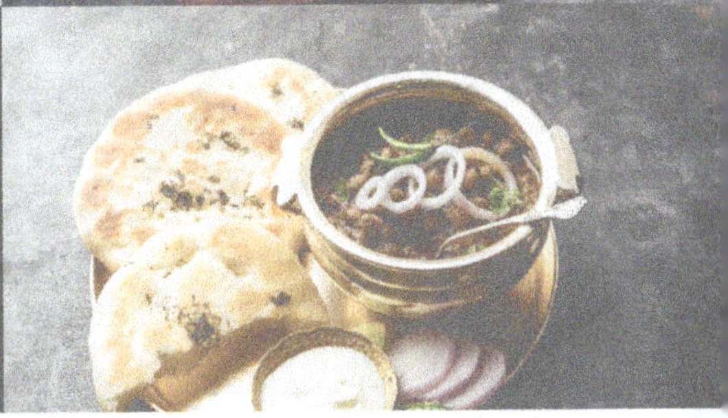

INTRODUCTION

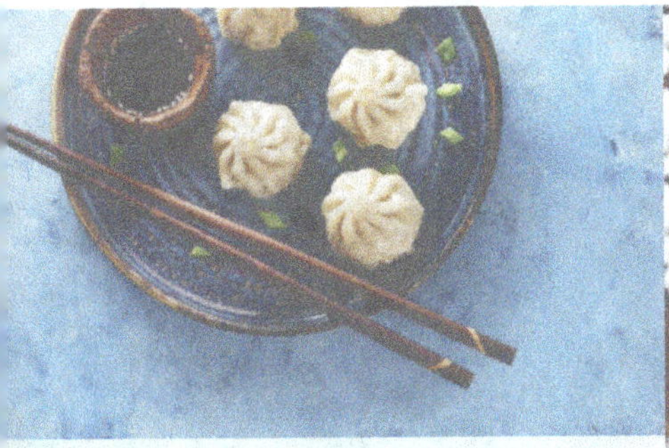

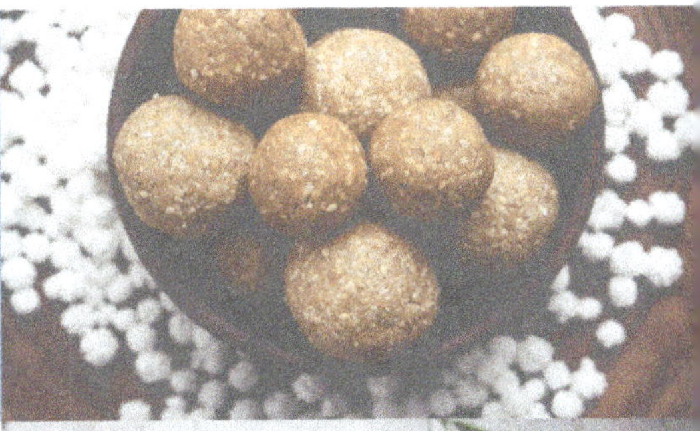

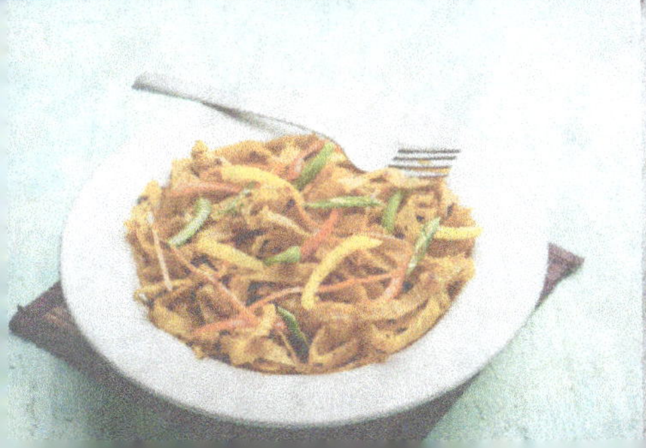

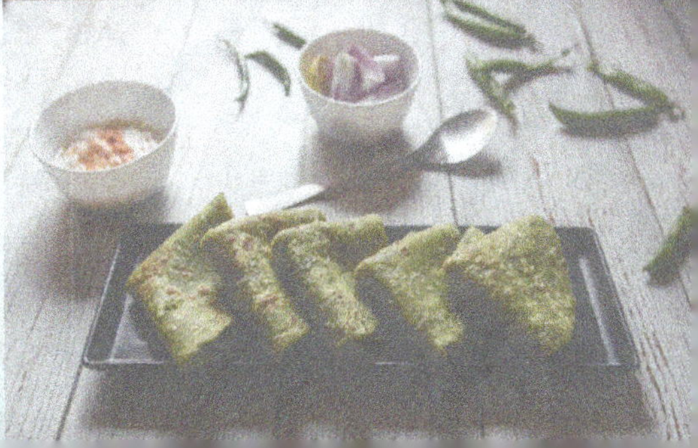

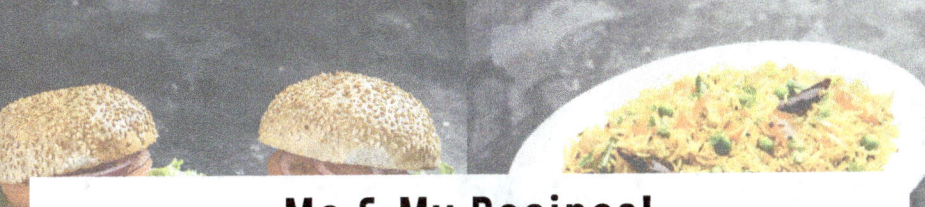

Me & My Recipes!

Hello, I am Dietitian Natasha Mohan and I have always strived to help people live healthy lives. I encountered many weight troubles myself.

From being overweight to now, encouraging people to live a healthy and nourished life. It's been a great challenge, but I never relinquished it. I aspire to encourage more people and help them overcome their weight challenges.

There are numerous benefits of healthy living and food. Healthy food can help you reduce the risk of severe disorders that are induced due to weight problems. And to balance your weight problems, these recipes are perfect. Many people come and question if they will be able to relish their favourite food in their weight loss journey. I always smile and say yes! At least with my healthy recipes, you can! Losing weight becomes so dull if you can't devour your favourite food. That's why I have brought to all of you my 50 impeccable recipes that you can incorporate into your busy lives and make the most of it.

My kitchen is my art studio, and instead of colours, I love to play with recipes. I love to recreate recipes. Recipes that are unhealthy, to make them healthy so you can enjoy them in your weight loss journey. This book includes 50 healthy and nourishing weight loss recipes.

Recipes for all your needs. Be it breakfast, lunch, dinner, or snack, along with beverages and as we know that everyone craves something sweet after their meals. That's why we have taken care of your sweet cravings too! All the recipes have measured calories. So, you can comfortably appreciate them in your journey. These recipes are healthful and effortless to make with ingredients available at home. So, you don't have to step out to make these, nor are these heavy on your pocket. So, try these incredible recipes and get a step closer to your weight loss goals and a healthy lifestyle.

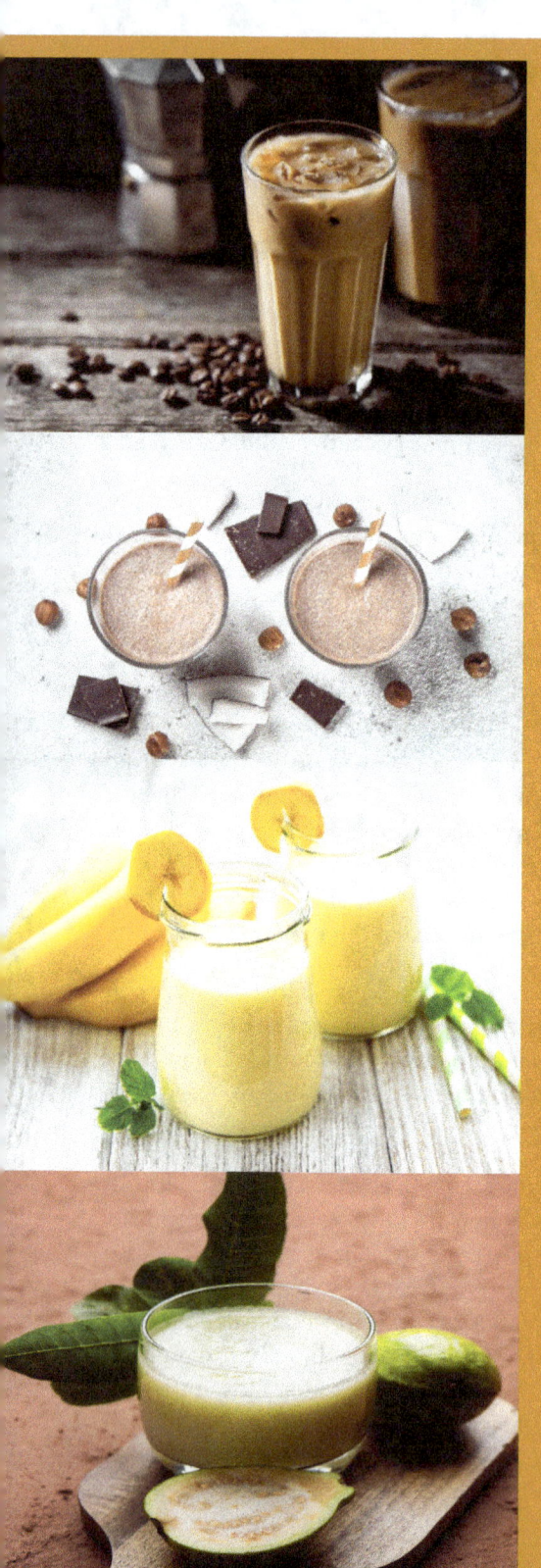

BEVERAGES

Did someone say smoothies? Are you looking out for some delectable smoothies and shake that don't provide any harm to your weight loss journey? You are at the right place! We know how hard it is to lose weight, and these killing summers call for some refreshing shakes and smoothies.

Who doesn't love frothy and creamy shakes or smoothies? Well, everyone does! But the fear of having them and gaining weight is very upsetting. So, to help you overcome this tension, we have brought for you all our fat-burning, low-in calories shake and smoothies' recipes. We have taken care of lactose intolerants too and workout lovers too. You can easily relish these in your weight loss journey without the fear of gaining weight, as they help in losing weight!

These are easy-to-make shakes and smoothies recipes that everyone can make. So now you don't have to ask your mothers or anyone to make some healthy and delicious smoothies or shakes for you as you can easily make them for yourselves. And the best part is you can relish these scrumptious smoothies shakes anytime. Be it your breakfast or you want something quick and energetic before your workout. You can take them! These are so filling that if you have them for your breakfast, you'll be good to go for the whole day or if you take them before your workout, you'll be filled with energy. You just have to follow the recipes step by step and you'll be fine!

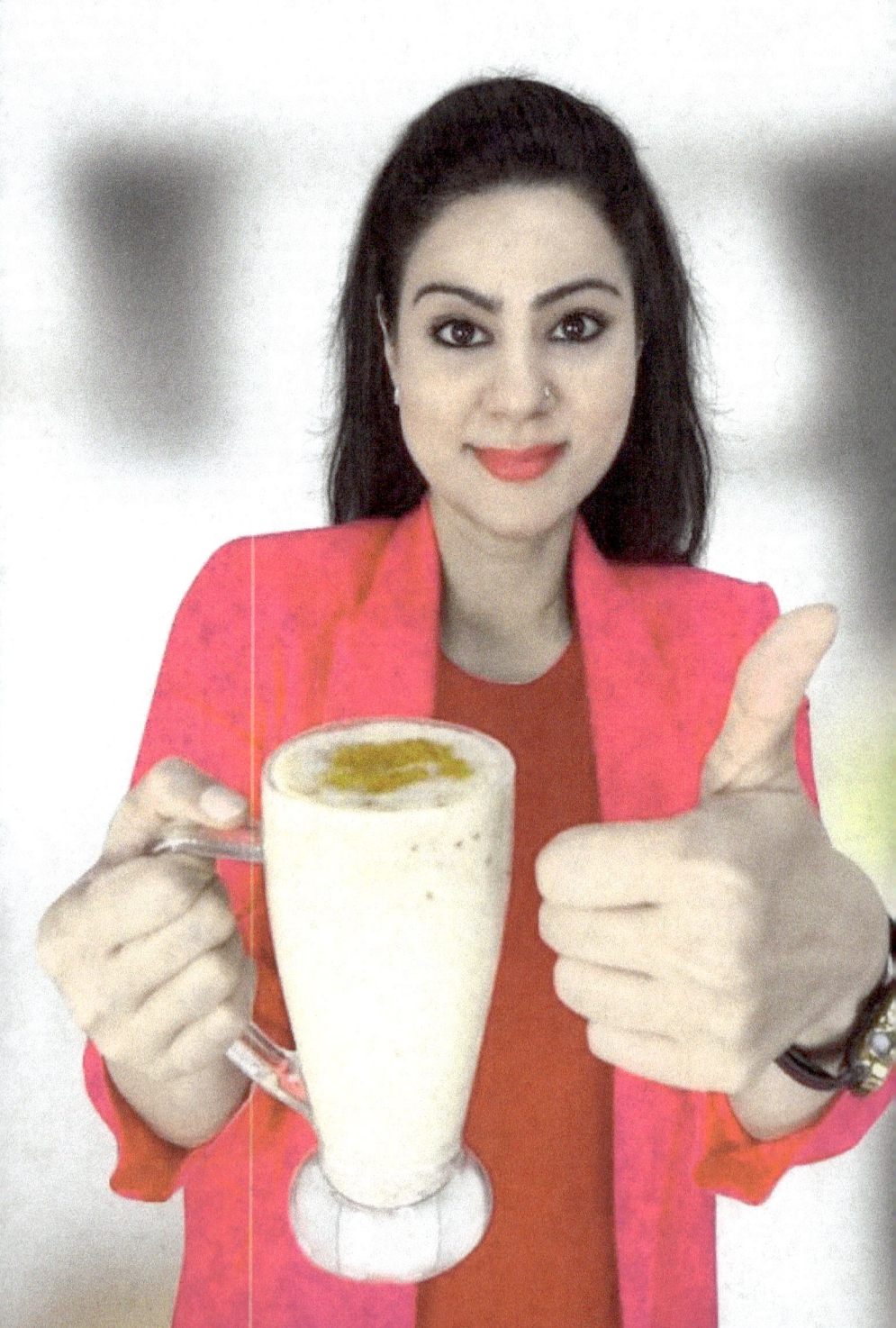

APPLE & OATS SMOOTHIE

Beat the summer heat with this quick and easy-to-make apple and oats smoothie. It's filled with the richness of apples and oats. A perfect beverage to relish in breakfast or snack time. It's only 249 calories!

INGREDIENTS:

- 1 diced apple
- 20 grams oats
- 4 pieces almonds (soaked and peeled) 1-piece pitted date 1/2 tsp cinnamon powder
- 100 ml skimmed milk

GARNISH:

- Cinnamon powder

DIRECTIONS:

1. In a blender, add the diced apple, 20 grams of oats powder, soaked almonds, and pitted date.

2. Next, add 1/2 tsp cinnamon powder, 100 ml skimmed milk and lots of ice. Blend until creamy and frothy.

3. Pour the smoothie into the glass and add 3-4 ice cubes.

4. Sprinkle some cinnamon powder to garnish, and, voilà, your apple and oats smoothie is ready. Enjoy!

BANANA SHAKE

Banana is everyone's favourite, but can you eat them during your weight loss journey? Of course, you can with this 175 calories recipe! This banana shake is low in calories but high in nutrients and provides you with instant energy and making it an ideal beverage for breakfast or your pre/post workout snack option.

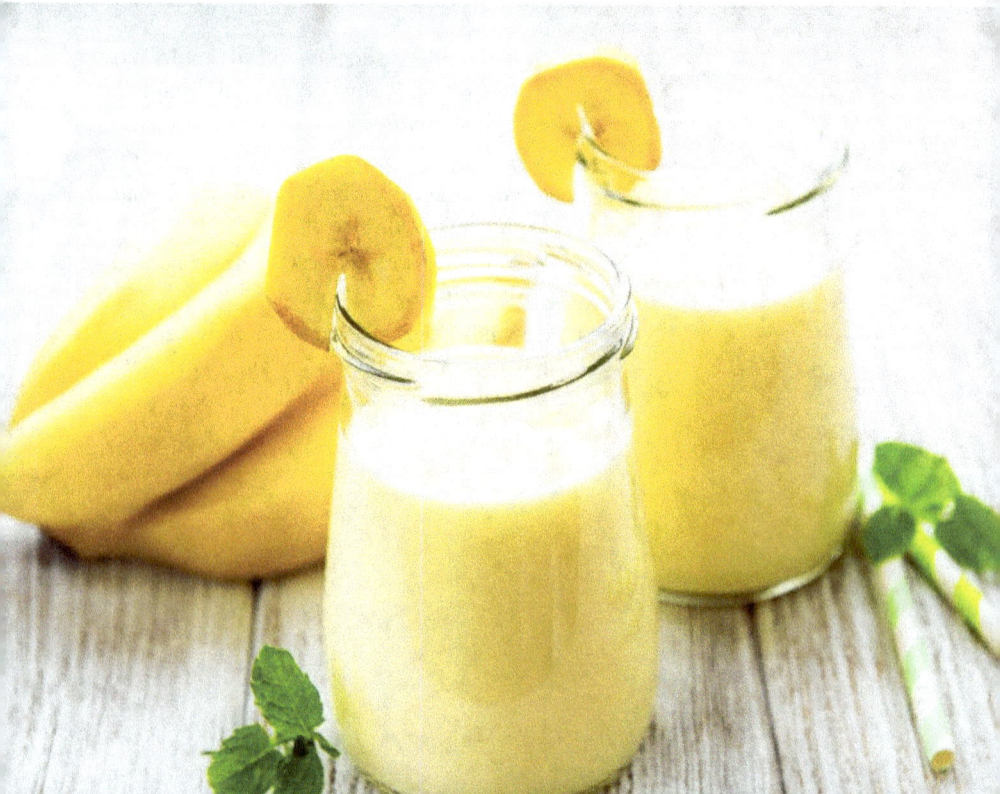

INGREDIENTS:

- 1 banana
- 20 grams oats powder
- 5-6 almonds (soaked and peeled)
- 1/2 tsp vanilla essence
- Approximately 1 glass of water

GARNISH:

- 1 tbsp soaked chia seeds.

DIRECTIONS:

1. In a blender, add banana, add oats powder and almonds to it.
2. Add 1/2 tsp vanilla essence and
3. approximately 1 glass of chilled water. Blend until smooth.
4. Next, take a glass and add lots of ice to it.
5. Pour the shake into the glass.
6. Add 1 tbsp soaked chia seeds and within minutes, your banana smoothie is ready. Enjoy!

Note:

Dry roast the oats and grind them to make oats powder.

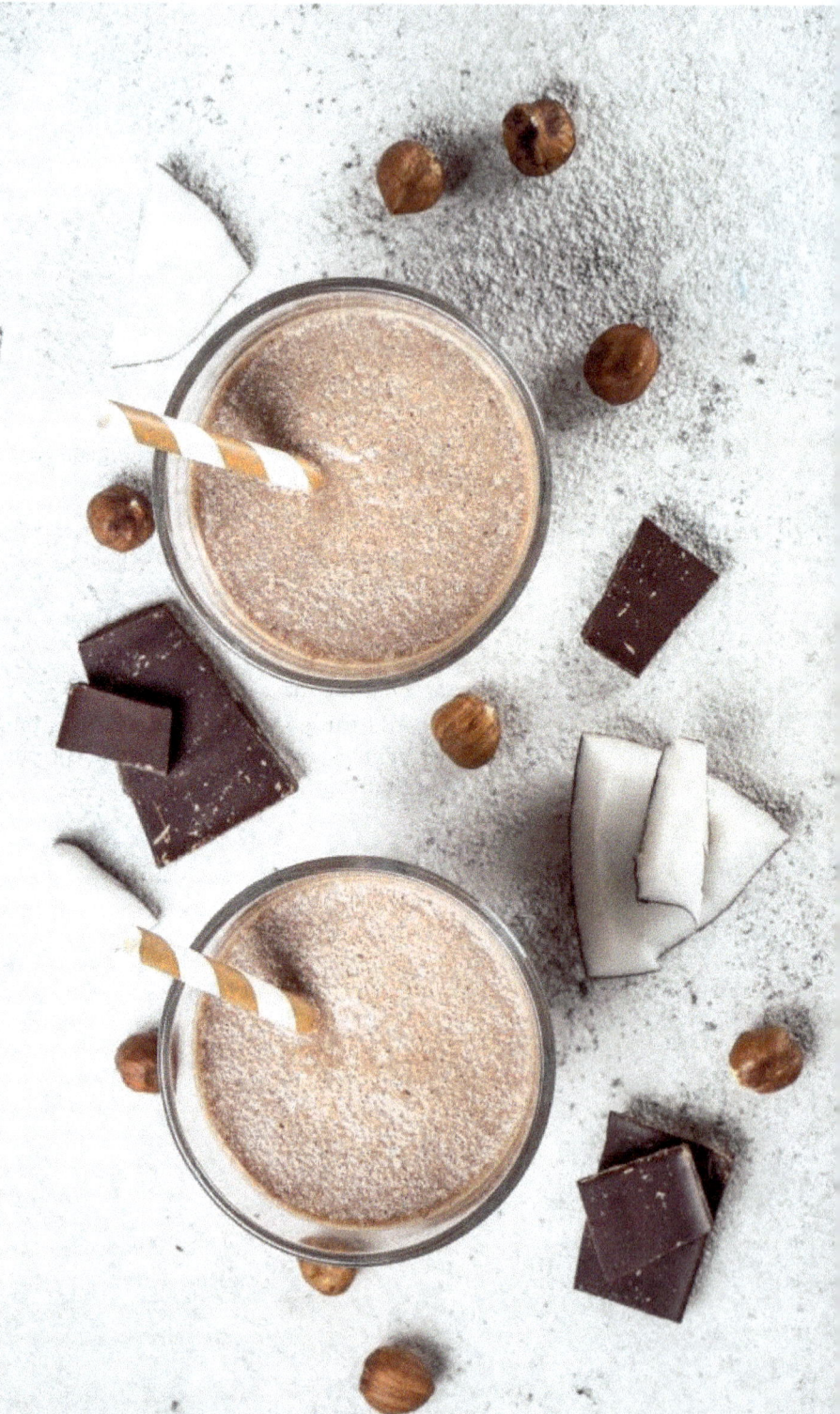

CHOCOLATE SMOOTHIE

Who does not like chocolate? But weight loss and chocolate don't match! So, we have brought you all this exciting chocolate smoothie recipe! It's so healthy yet scrumptious that your kids will love it too! You can devour it in the morning or evening. And the best part is it only contains 150 calories!

INGREDIENTS:

- 30 grams chopped coconut
- 1 tbsp cocoa powder (unsweetened)
- 2 tbsp oats powder*
  Approximately 1 tsp vanilla essence
- Approximately 1 glass of water

GARNISH:

- Cocoa powder

DIRECTIONS:

1. In a blender, add coconut pieces, 1 tbsp unsweetened cocoa powder, 2 tbsp oats powder, and 1 tsp vanilla essence.
2. Add a lot of ice cubes and approximately 1 glass of water.
3. Blend it for 2-3 minutes until smooth because coconut takes time to blend.
4. You'll get a frothy mixture. Pour the mixture into a glass with lots of ice.
5. Sprinkle some cocoa powder to garnish it and enjoy!

Note:

Dry roast the oats and grind them to make oats powder.

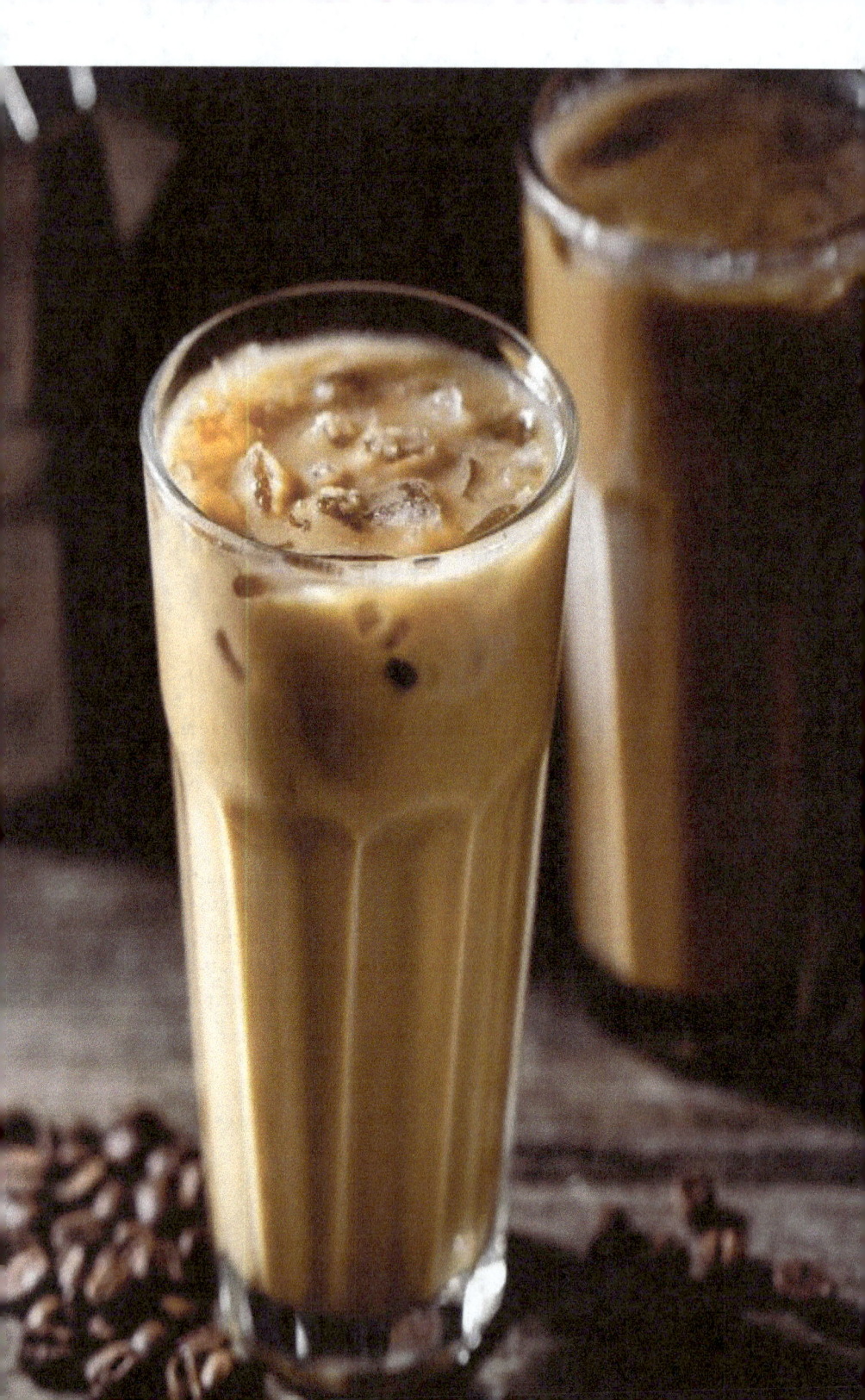

COLD COFFEE

For all the coffee lovers out there, this recipe is a must-try! Only 138 calories of cold coffee. You will love it! Once you try this recipe, you will forget about every other.

You can easily incorporate this into your weight loss journey.

INGREDIENTS:

- 1.5 tsp cocoa powder
- 1.5 tsp coffee powder
- 2 tbsp oats powder
- 1 tsp stevia
- 1/2 glass chilled water

GARNISH:

- Chocolate sauce (optional)
- Grated chocolate

DIRECTIONS:

1. In a blender, add 1.5 tsp cocoa powder, 1.5 tsp coffee powder, 2 tbsp oats powder, stevia, and 1/2 glass of chilled water.
2. Add a lot of ice and blend until creamy.
3. Take a glass and apply chocolate sauce over it.
4. Add lots of ice cubes and pour the coffee into the glass.
5. Sprinkle some grated chocolate over it, and voila, your cold coffee is ready. Enjoy!

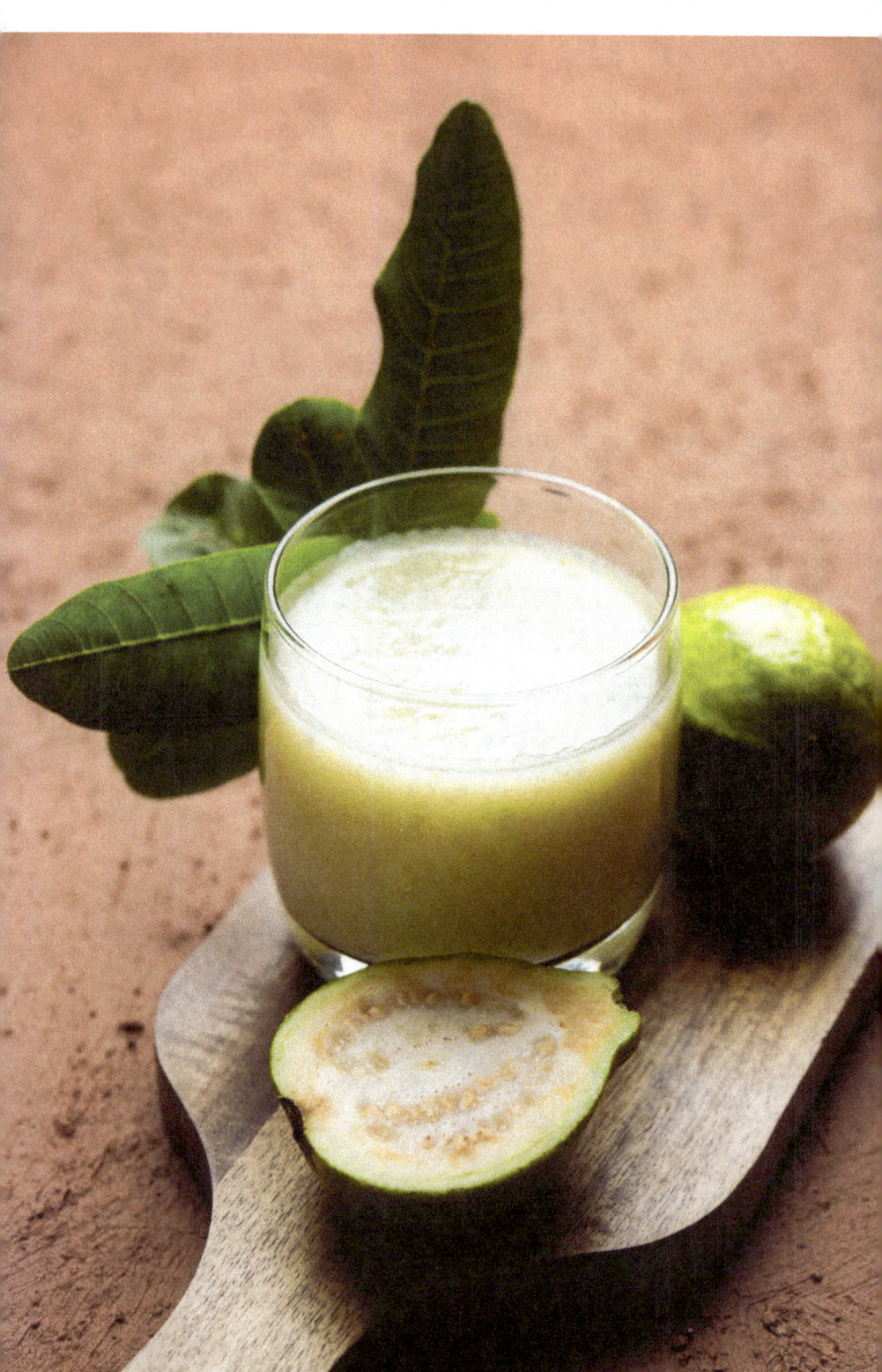

GUAVA MOJITO

The summer definitely calls for something light and refreshing. Here we are with Natasha Mohan's amazing guava mojito recipe. So light, so refreshing! It's a perfect beverage for all occasions and it contains only 100 calories!

INGREDIENTS:

- 1 guava (seedless)
- 1/2 tsp black salt
- 1/2 tsp red chilli powder
- 1 tsp flaxseeds
- 1/2 tsp cumin seeds
- Half lemon

GARNISH:

- Mint leaves

DIRECTIONS:

1. In a blender, add chopped seedless guava, black salt, red chilli powder, flaxseeds, cumin seeds and lemon juice.
2. Add a lot of ice cubes, a little water if required and blend it.
3. Take a glass, add ice cubes to it and pour the guava smoothie into it.
4. Garnish with some mint leaves and enjoy!

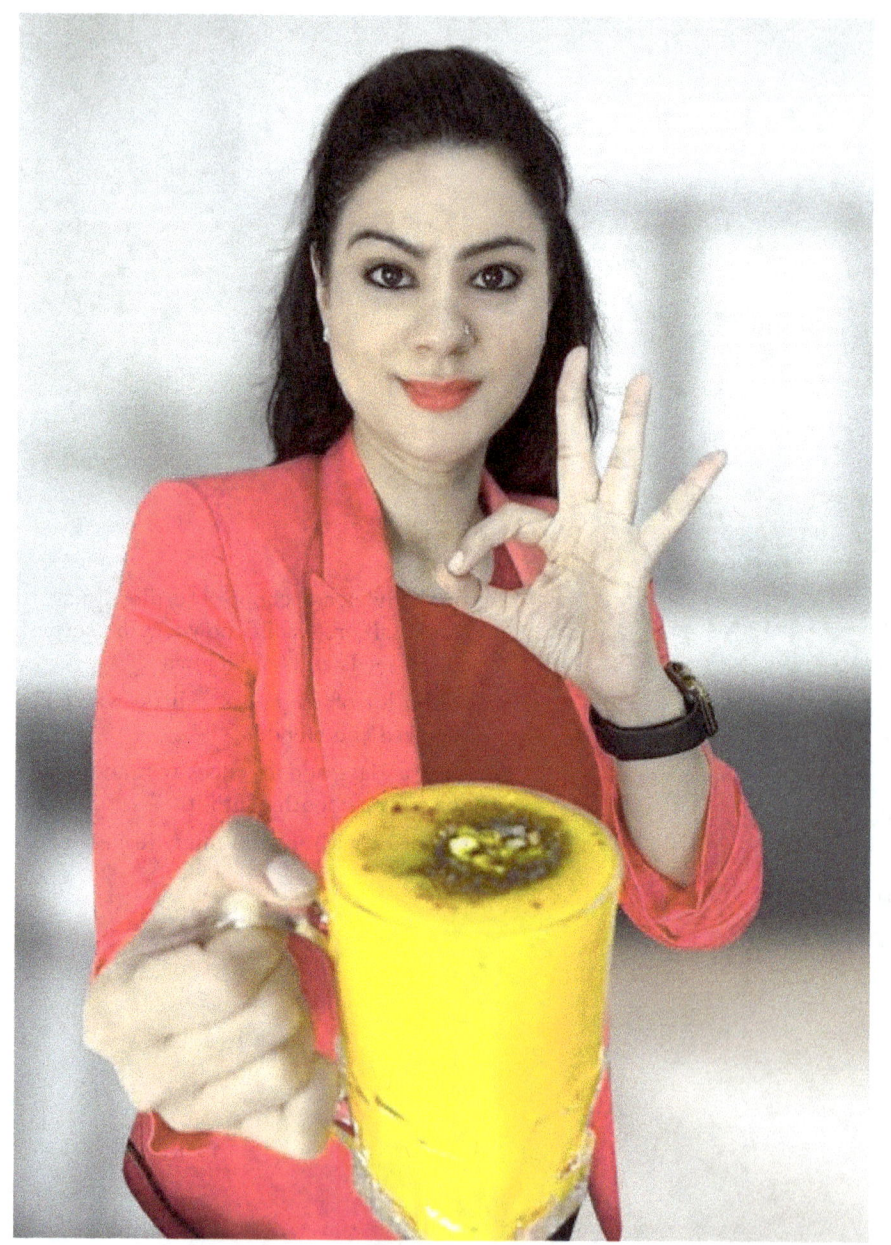

MANGO SHAKE

Everyone loves mango but, cannot relish it due to the weight stress. But, with this mango shake recipe, you can enjoy your favourite mangoes even when trying to lose weight because it contains only 120 calories. It's very healthy and nutritious.

INGREDIENTS:

- 100 grams chopped mango
- 1/2 glass skimmed milk
- 1/2 glass water

GARNISH:

- 2-3 pieces of pistachios (unsalted)
- 1 tbsp soaked chia seeds

DIRECTIONS:

1. In a blender, add chopped mangoes, 1/2 glass of skimmed milk and 1/2 glass of water to it.
2. Add lots of ice to it and blend until smooth.
3. Take a glass, add 2-3 ice cubes, and pour the mango shake into it.
4. Garnish your mango shake with chopped pistachios and chia seeds.
5. Serve it chilled, and enjoy!

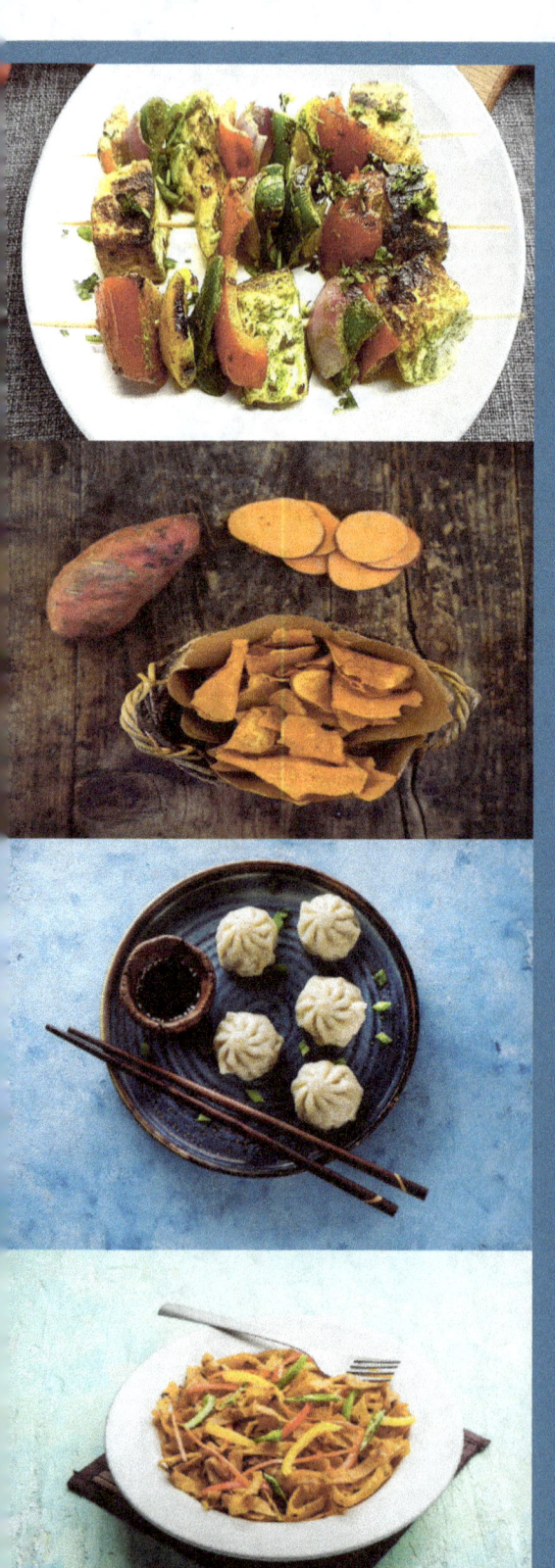

SNACKS

Evening time is the most strenuous time for a person trying to lose weight. Many people fail at this time only. They try and work so hard the whole day or even skip their meals but often get hungry at this time and lose control over what they eat. It's the most crucial and dangerous time. As it's the time after you have had your meals and you feel hungry and don't know what to eat. So, you end up eating junk food that makes you gain weight.

Junk food is your worst enemy when you're trying to lose weight as it's full of oil and preservatives. So instead of snacking on junk food, snack on something healthy. Food that is not only nourishing but helps you lose weight too.

We all feel hungry at this time and crave something that we cannot resist. We look for something that is filling and satisfies our cravings for junk food. So, what if we say that we have got all the taste but in a healthy way? Food that tastes the same as junk food but is more wholesome than theirs. Don't believe us? Try for yourselves then! We have brought for you all our startling snack recipes, which are not only healthy but mouth-watering too. These have all food that you love to snack on evening time. Be it your favourite momos, crispy chips, noodles, samosa, chaats, bhel puri and all your preferred food. We have brought you all.

So now, you don't have to spend money on junk food items instead can make yourself the healthy version of them at your home. Our recipes are not only nutritious but are pocket friendly too. You can comfortably cook these and satisfy all your junk food cravings without eating junk food. So, what are you waiting for? Try these now and snack smartly with us!

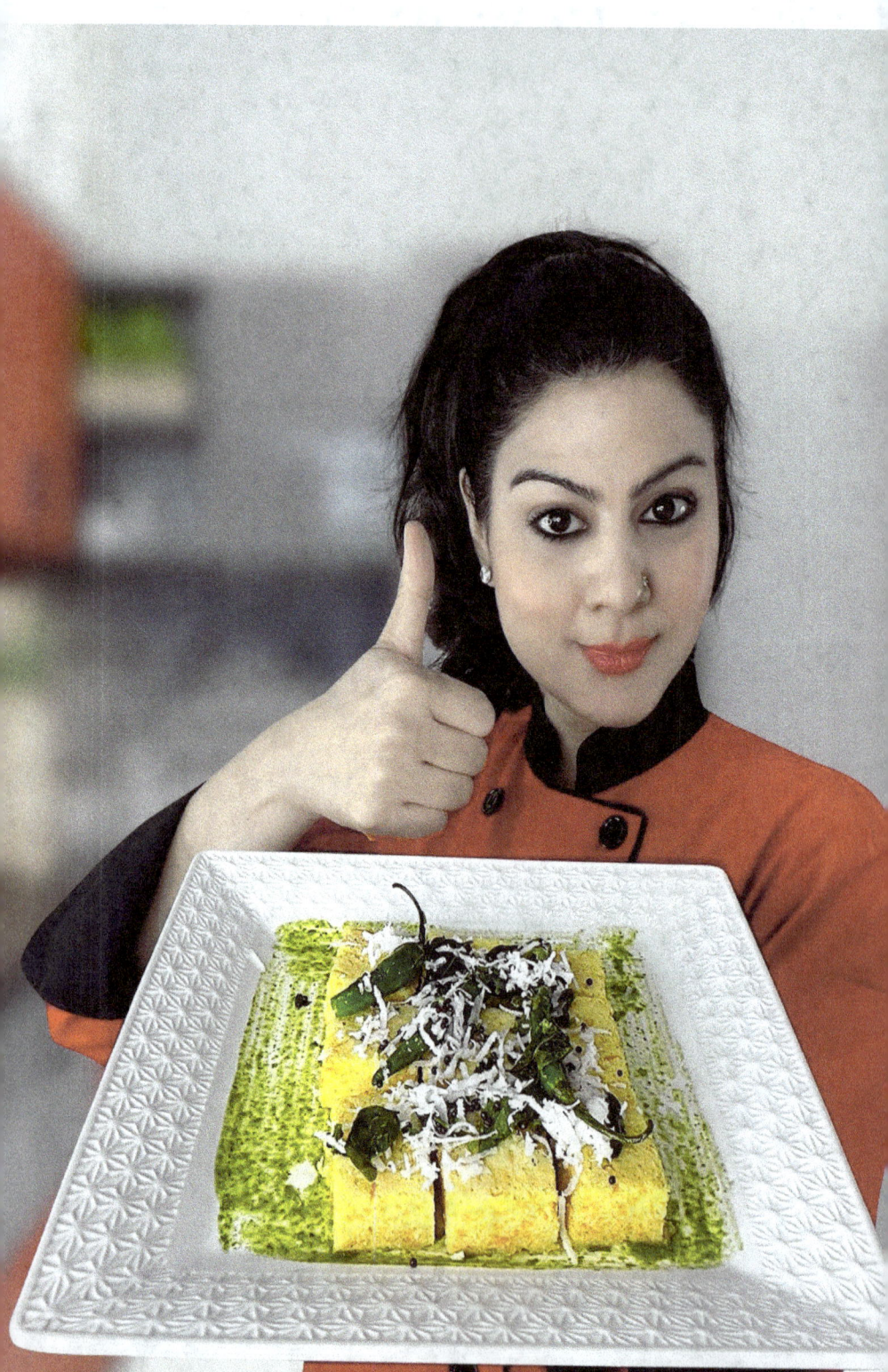

MOONG DAL DHOKLA

Sometimes in dieting, you get cravings that you can't resist and one of them is dhokla. So, to satisfy your craving here's our version of slim-waist moong dal dhokla which contains only 30 calories per piece. You can easily enjoy this in your weight loss journey without any stress.

INGREDIENTS:

- 1 cup moong dal (overnight soaked)
- Salt according to your taste
- 1 cup grated carrot
- 1/2 tsp eno
- 1 tsp oil
- 1/2 tsp mustard seeds
- 1 tbsp curry leaves
- 1 tbsp finely chopped coriander leaves
- 4-5 green chillies
- Water

GARNISH:

- Grated coconut

Note:

Use a toothpick to check if the dhokla is cooked or not. Take the toothpick, put it in the dhokla, and check if it's clear or not. If it's clear, then the dhokla Is cooked. Otherwise, let it cook for more minutes.

DIRECTIONS:

1. For dhokla batter, Soak 1 cup moong dal overnight. Next, rinse and add it to a blender.
2. Add some salt and blend until smooth.
3. Transfer the paste into a bowl. Take a hand blender and blend it until fluffy.
4. Next, add 1 cup grated carrot to the paste and mix it with light hands. Then, add 1/2 tsp ENO to it. Mix it well.
5. Now take a mould and grease it with little oil and transfer entire the batter to it.
6. Steam it for about 5-10 minutes in a steamer until cooked properly. *
7. For dhokla tempering, in a pan, add 1 tsp oil, mustard seeds, curry leaves, and green chillies. Cook until mustard seeds start to crackle on a low flame.
8. Next, add chopped coriander leaves, a pinch of salt and some water to it.
9. Cut the dhokla into pieces and pour this tempering all over it.
10. Garnish it with some grated coconut and enjoy!

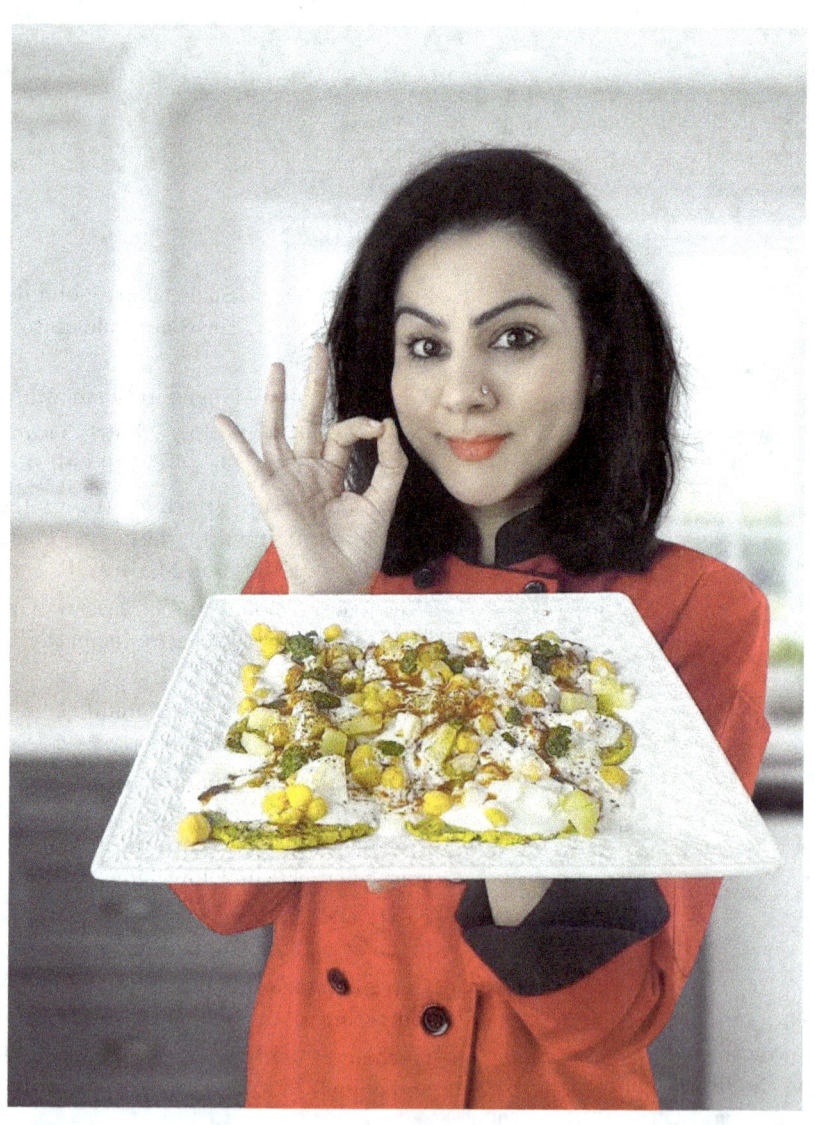

CHATPATI CHAAT

Why go out to eat chatpati chaat when you can easily make one at your home? Make the most delicious and healthy chatpati chaat at home that makes you and your family happy with the ingredients easily available at home. And it's only 28 calories per piece!

INGREDIENTS:

- 2 tbsp gram flour Water
- 1/2 tsp cumin seeds
- 1 tsp chopped green chillies
- 1 tsp carom seeds
- 1/4 tsp asafoetida (hing)
- 1-2 tbsp chopped spinach leaves
- Oil (for cooking)
- 20 grams boiled chickpeas
- 20 grams finely chopped onion (optional)
- 20 grams boiled potato
- 1 bowl curd
- 1 tsp stevia
- green chutney
- Imli and dates chutney

GARNISH:

- Red chilli powder
- Raw mango powder

DIRECTIONS:

1. In a bowl, add gram flour and water to make a paste. It should not be too thick or too watery. Whisk well and make sure no lumps are left.
2. Next, add cumin seeds, green chillies, carom seeds, and asafoetida. Mix the ingredients well.
3. Now, add spinach leaves and mix all ingredients well.
4. Take a non-stick pan, apply a little oil, and spread the batter using a tsp. Try to spread the batter as thin as possible. Cook until crunchy from both sides.
5. Transfer the gram and spinach papdi to the plate and add boiled chickpeas, onions, and boiled potatoes over it.
6. Now, take a bowl of curd and mix 1 tsp of stevia to make it sweet.
7. Now, spread curd over all the ingredients.
8. Next, drizzle green chutney and imli (Tamarind) and dates chutney.
9. Garnish it with some red chilli powder and raw mango powder and enjoy!

GUILT-FREE MOMOS

Every child's favourite and mother's biggest enemy momos! But not anymore! Try this exciting guilt-free momos recipe that you'll love, and your kids will love too. Filled with veggies! The perfect way to fulfil your family's vegetable requirement. And yes you can relish momos in your weight loss journey with this recipe! It's only 40 calories per momo. Enjoy!

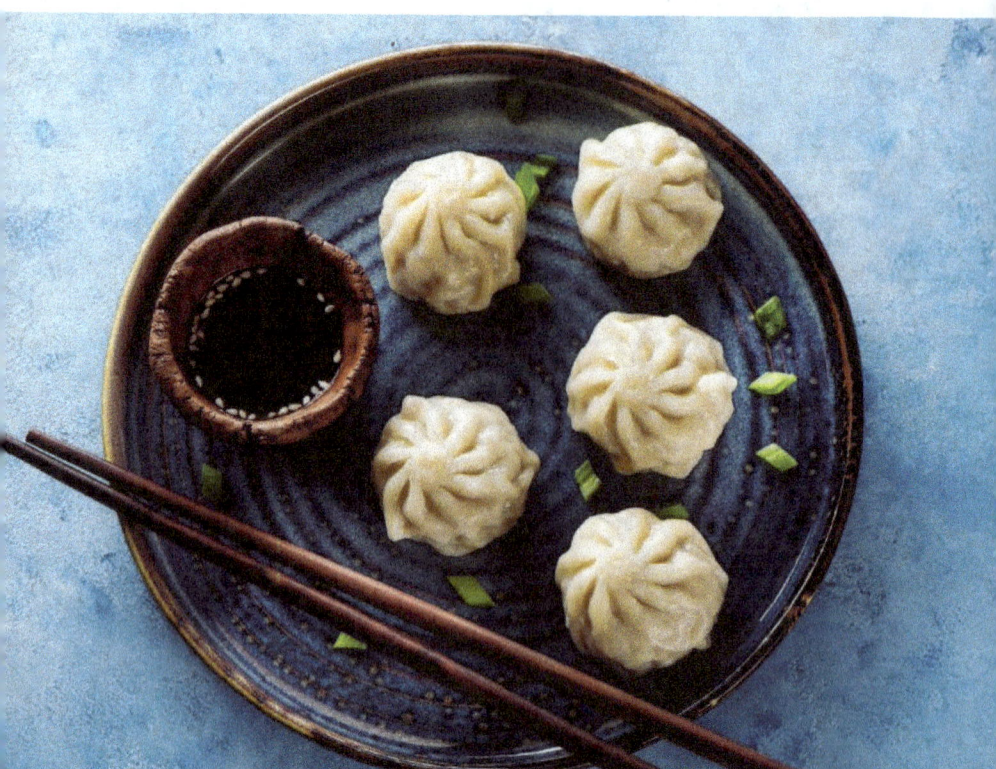

INGREDIENTS:

- 1/2 cup grated cabbage
- 1/4 cup finely chopped onion
- 1/4 cup grated carrot
- 1 tsp finely chopped green chillies
- 10-15 finely chopped coriander leaves
- 1 tsp white pepper powder
- 1 tsp garlic paste
- Salt according to your taste
- 1/2 tsp soy sauce
- 1/2 tsp red chilli sauce
- Wheat flour (atta)
- 1/2 tbsp ghee

DIRECTIONS:

1. To make the filling of momos, take a bowl and add cabbage, onions, carrots, green chillies, and coriander leaves to it.

2. Next, add white pepper powder, garlic paste, salt, soy sauce and red chilli sauce. Mix it well.

3. To make the dough, take a bowl and add wheat flour, water, salt and a little oil. Knead it properly. Don't keep the dough too hard.

4. Take small balls of dough and roll them as thin as possible.

5. Put the momos filling inside and give them momo shape.

6. Steam the momos for about 10 minutes.

7. After steaming the momos, take a pan and spread a little oil over it and lightly roast the momos. Or you can have them in the steamed form too. Enjoy!

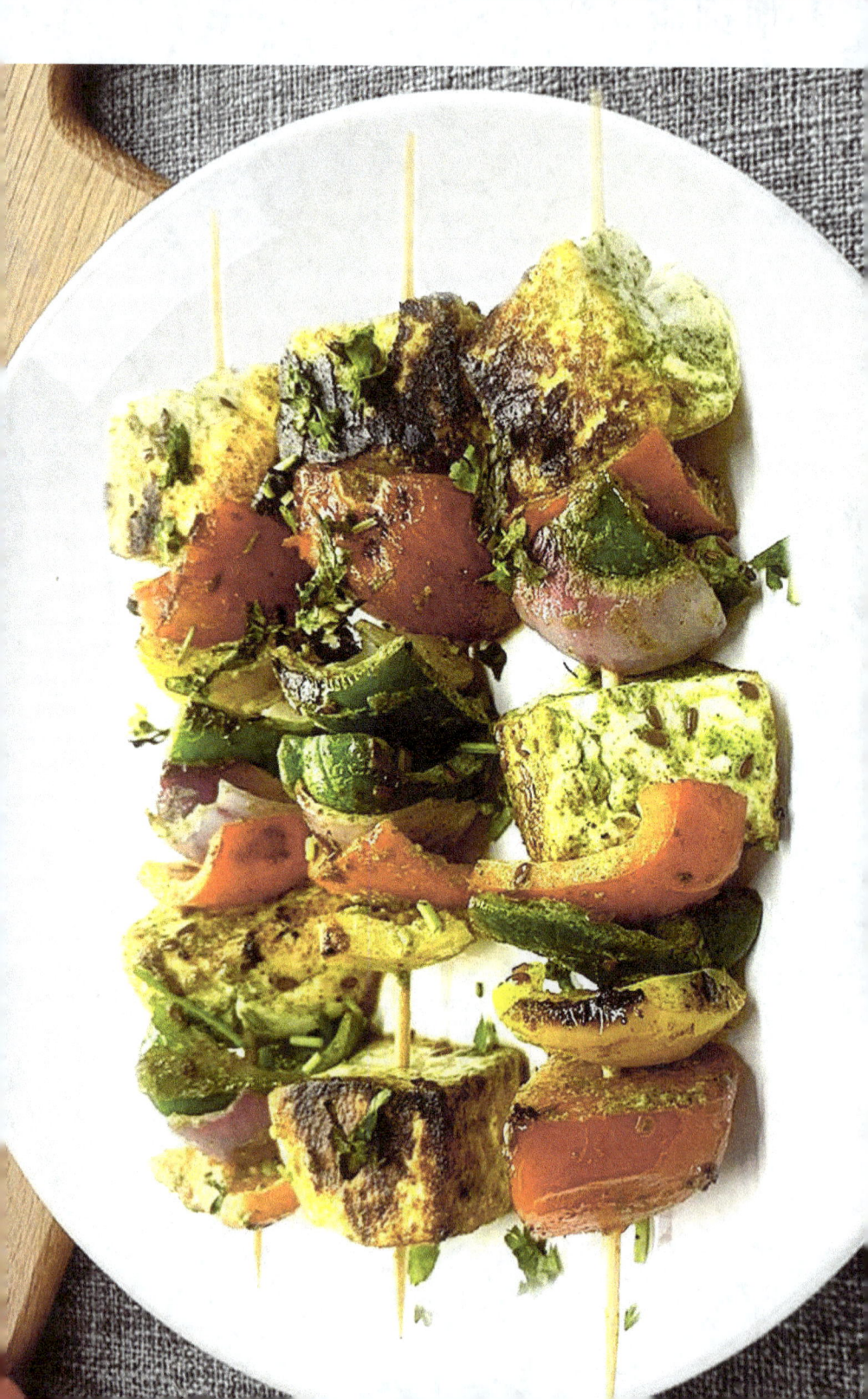

PANEER TIKKA

Craving some crispy paneer tikka but afraid to gain weight? Not anymore! Try this amazing paneer tikka recipe and satisfy all your cravings and hunger. This scrumptious recipe contains only 360 calories.

INGREDIENTS:

- 5-6 coriander leaves
- 5-6 mint leaves
- 3-4 whole green chillies
- 1 tsp garlic paste
- Half Lemon
- 1/2 cup curd
- 1 tsp coriander powder
- 1/2 tsp cumin powder
- 1/2 tsp garam masala
- 1/2 raw mango powder
- Salt according to your taste
- 1 tbsp roughly chopped each bell pepper (red, yellow)
- 1 tbsp roughly chopped onion
- 1 tbsp roughly chopped tomato
- 100 grams paneer (Chopped into cubes)
- 1/2 tbsp oil
- 1 tbsp flaxseeds

DIRECTIONS:

1. For paneer's marination, take a blender and put coriander leaves, mint leaves, green chillies, garlic paste, lemon juice, and curd. Blend it properly until it's smooth.

2. Next, take the mixture out and add coriander powder, raw mango powder, garam masala, cumin powder, and salt. Mix all the ingredients well.

3. Next, add roughly chopped bell peppers, tomatoes, and onions to the mixture.

4. Now, add paneer cubes and mix them well into the mixture. Keep it in the refrigerator for about 1-2 hours.

5. Assemble the paneer cubes and vegetables into a skewer. If you don't have it, you can directly place them onto a pan.

6. Take a pan and apply some oil to it, and put the paneer skewers in.

7. Grill them well till they get cooked and crispy from both sides, and sprinkle 1 tbsp flaxseeds.

8. Take the paneer skewers out of the pan. Garnish with some coriander and mint leaves, and enjoy!

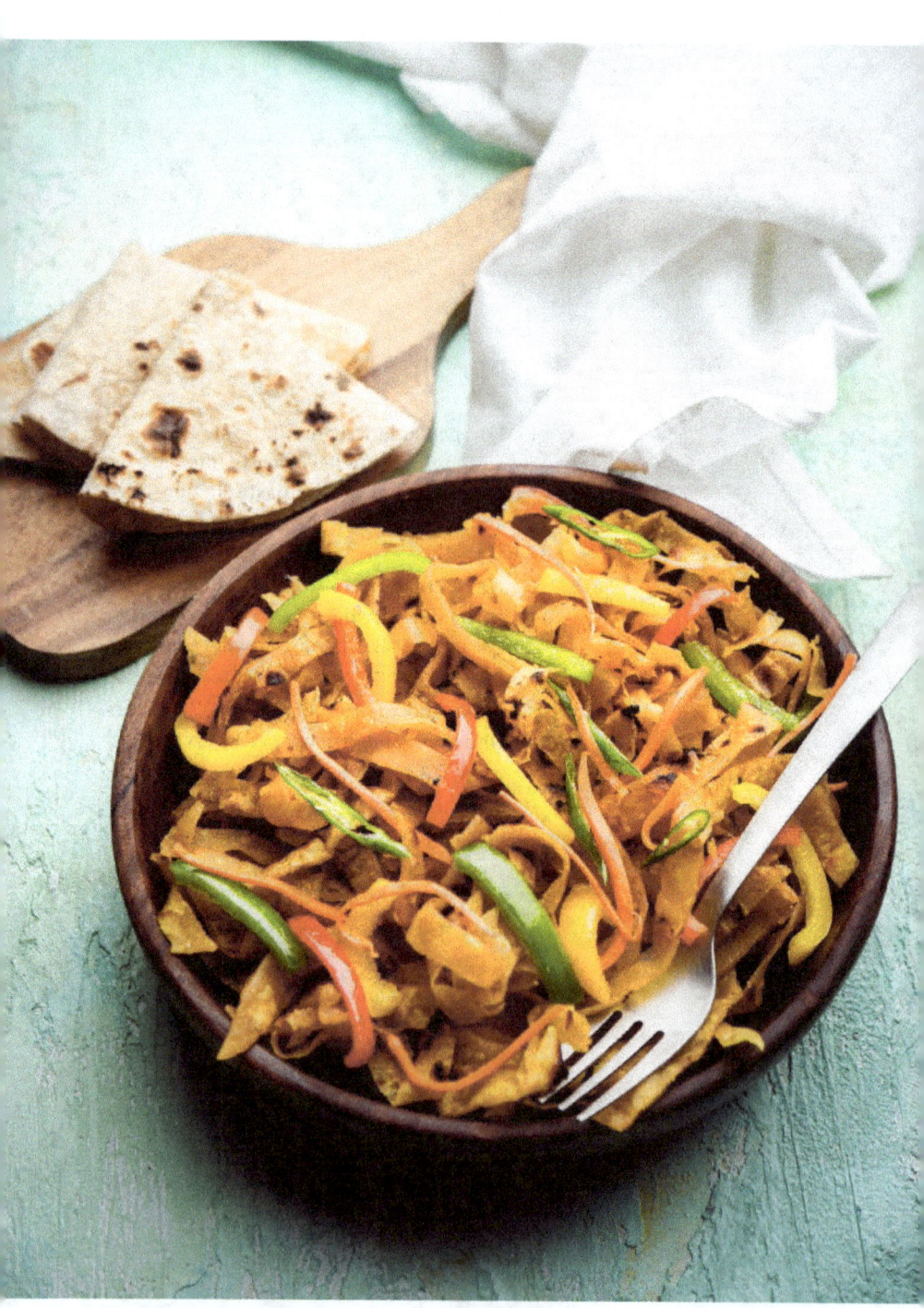

ROTI NOODLES

Noodle in weight loss, seems impossible right? Try Natasha Mohan's roti noodles recipe that will give you full desi-chowmein vibes with a healthy twist! And it's only 128 calories!

INGREDIENTS:

- 2 leftover rotis (thin slices)
- 1 tbsp oil
- 1 tsp mustard seeds
- 2 tbsp onions (julienne)
- 2 tbsp carrots (julienne)
- 2 tbsp green capsicum (julienne)
- 2 tbsp red and yellow bell pepper (julienne)
- Salt according to your taste
- 1/2 tsp black pepper powder
- 1/2 tsp raw mango powder (amchur)

DIRECTIONS:

1. Take 2 rotis, roll them and slice them thinly. Give them the shape of noodles.

2. Next, take a pan and add oil to it. Let it heat for 2 minutes.

3. Add mustard seeds, onions, carrots, bell peppers and green capsicum to the pan. Sauté the vegetables for approximately 2-3 minutes.

4. Add roti noodles to the pan and mix them well with vegetables.

5. Now add salt, black pepper powder, and raw mango powder to the noodles. Mix the ingredients well.

6. Serve the noodles hot, and enjoy!

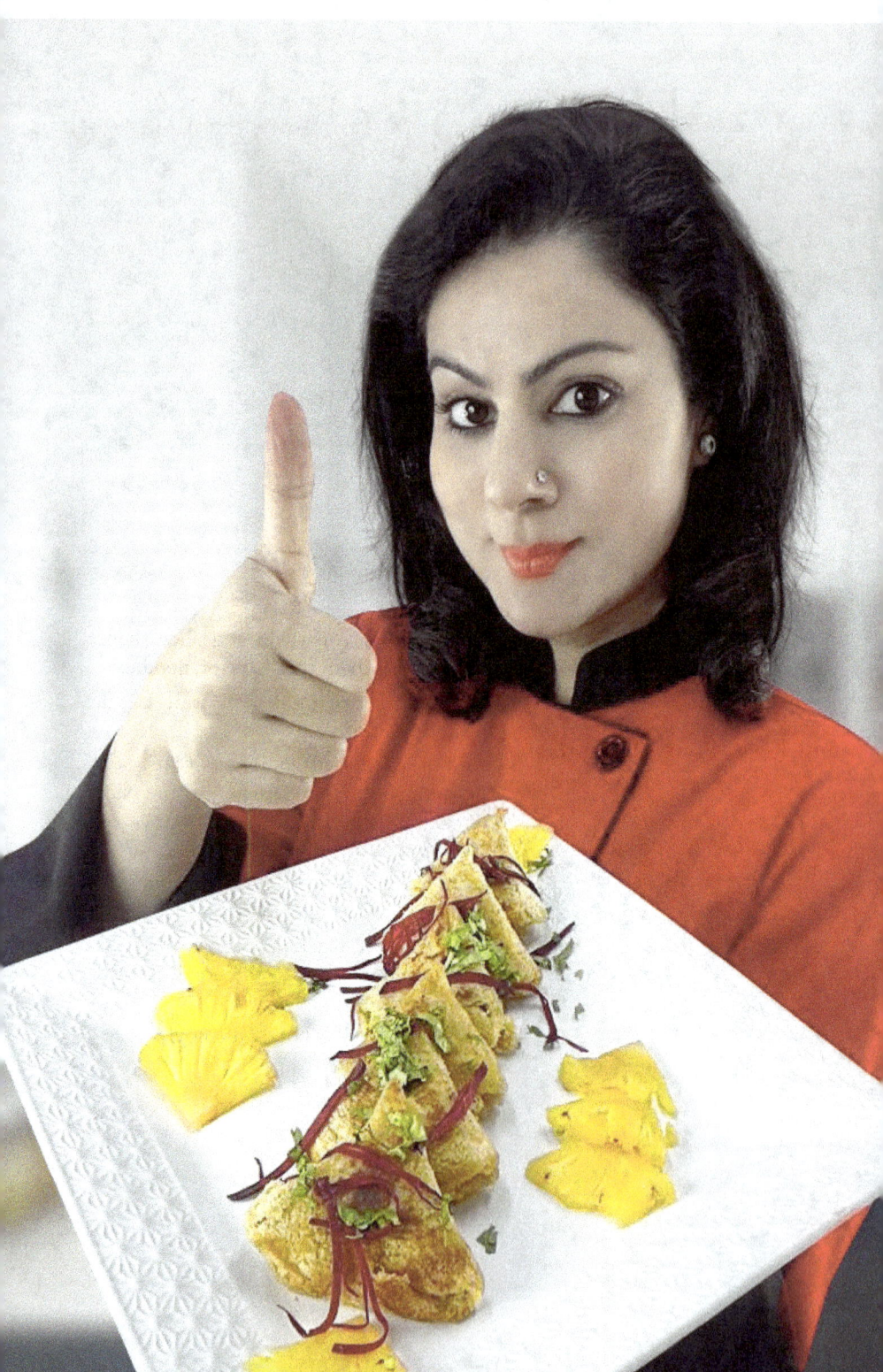

SAMOSA

No one knows how to say no to a samosa! Everyone loves crispy and crunchy samosa, especially during teatime. But can you enjoy it without the tension of gaining weight? Yes, with this recipe you can! Because it's only 45 calories per piece of samosa. You can include this in your weight loss journey and relish it as an evening snack!

INGREDIENTS:

- 1 tsp oil
- 1/2 tsp cumin seeds
- 1/4 tsp coriander seeds
- 1/2 tsp grated ginger
- 1-1.5 tbsp small paneer cubes
- 1-1.5 tbsp boiled peas
- Salt according to your taste
- 1 tsp raw mango powder (amchur)
- 1/2 tsp coriander powder
- 1/4 tsp red chilli powder
- Atta bread

DIRECTIONS:

1. In a frying pan, add 1 tsp of oil, cumin seeds, coriander seeds, and grated ginger. Sauté it for 2 minutes until it starts to crackle.
2. Next, add paneer cubes and boiled peas.
3. Now, add salt, coriander powder, raw mango powder, and red chilli powder. Cook for 3-4 minutes on low flame until the paneer is roasted.
4. Take 1 atta bread, cut its edges and with the help of a roller, roll it thin. Now, cut the bread into triangular halves and apply water over it.
5. Join one corner of the bread half with the other one and give it a samosa shape.
6. Fill the paneer filling inside the bread. Join it with the help of water.
7. Now, take a frying pan and lightly brush some oil on it. Put the samosa in the pan and cook until it turns brown and crispy.
8. Garnish them with chopped coriander leaves and some thinly chopped beetroot slices and enjoy!

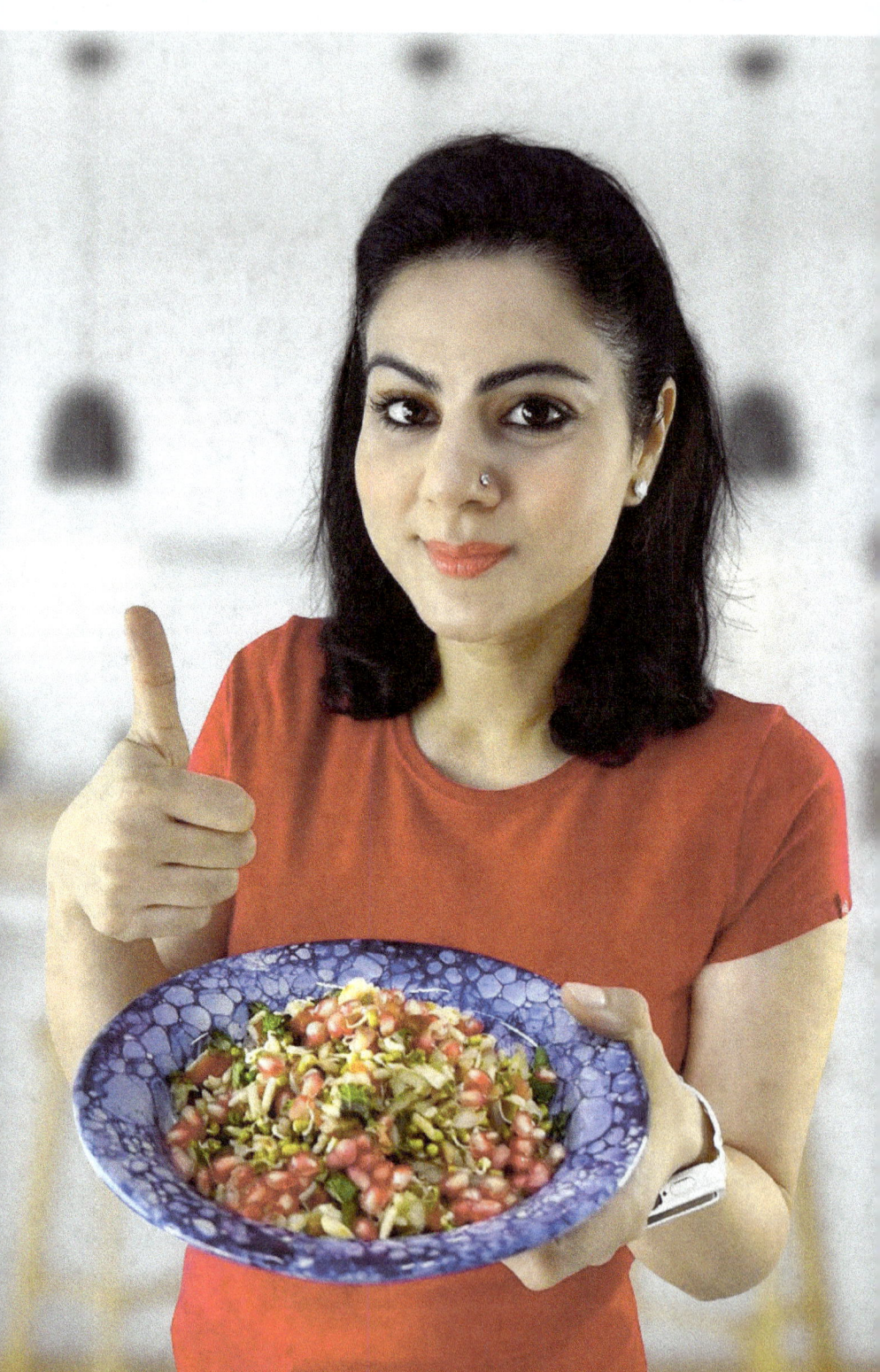

SPROUTS BHEL PURI

Looking for something crunchy to snack on? Well, we have got you covered! Try this light yet protein-filled bhel puri recipe. It will help you satisfy your hunger and keep you fuller for longer. And it's less than 150 calories!

INGREDIENTS:

- 50 grams washed sprouts (not boiled)
- 1 tbsp finely chopped onion
- 1 tbsp finely chopped tomato
- 1 tbsp finely chopped cucumber
- 1/2 tbsp finely chopped coriander leaves
- 1-2 tsp chopped green chillies
- Salt according to your taste
- 1 tsp black pepper powder
- 1 tbsp dry roasted peanuts (unsalted)
- 1 tsp green chutney
- 1 tsp date & imly chutney (homemade)
- 5-6 mint leaves
- 20 grams murmura

GARNISH:

- Pomegranate seeds

DIRECTIONS:

1. In a bowl add washed sprouts, finely chopped onions, tomatoes, cucumber, green chillies, and coriander leaves.
2. Now, add salt, black pepper powder, roasted peanuts, green chutney, and imly chutney.
3. Next, take some mint leaves, break them, and add and mix all the ingredients properly.
4. Now, add murmura. Always add murmura in the end so that it stays crunchy when you eat it.
5. Garnish your bhel puri with some pomegranate seeds and enjoy!

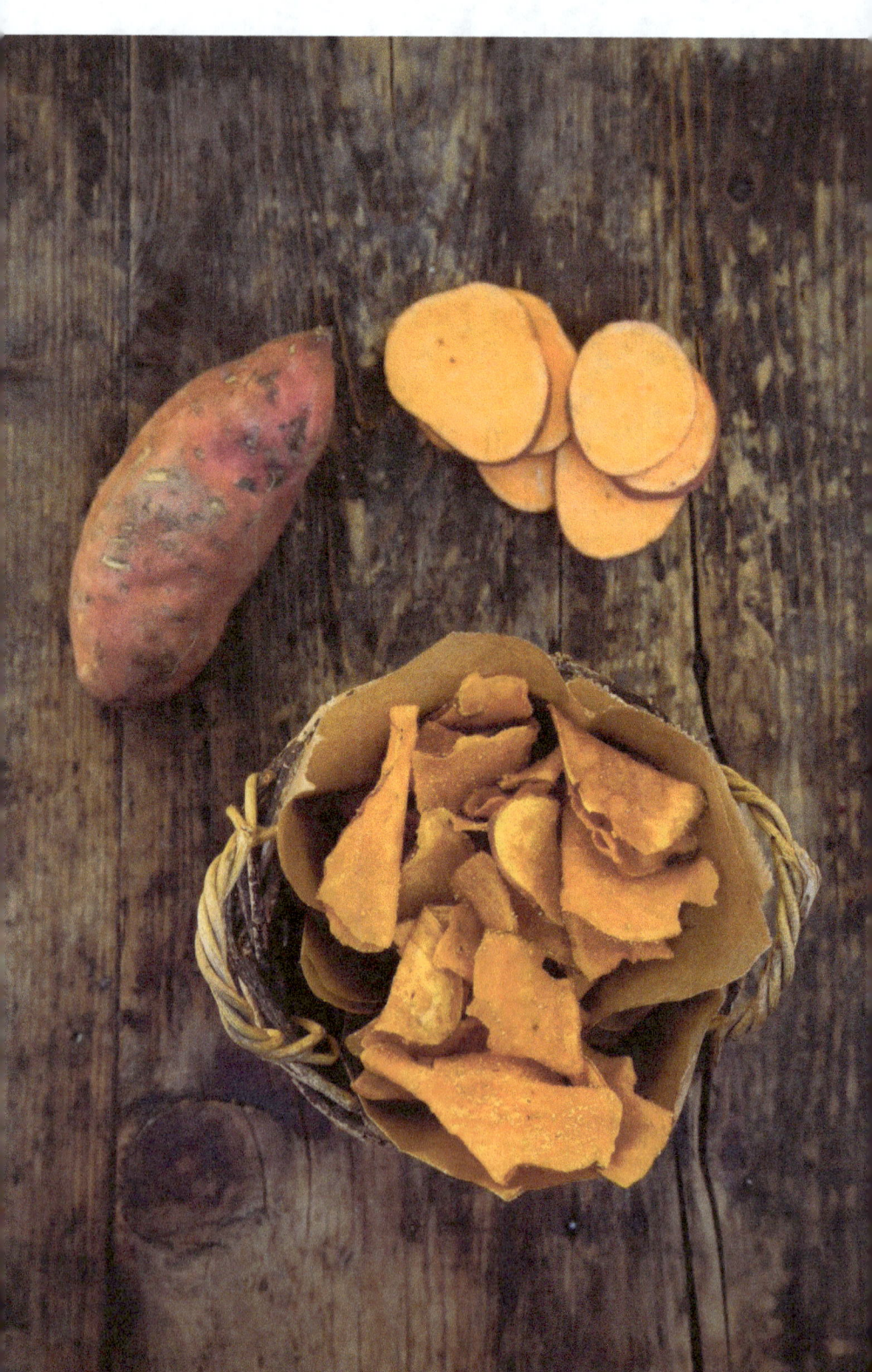

SWEET POTATO CHIPS

Cannot stop munching on unhealthy packed chips? No, worries! We have got your back! Try our amazing sweet potato chips recipe that is not only delicious but so healthy that you can munch on them without any stress of gaining weight! And it's only 3 calories per piece! So, relish them comfortably.

INGREDIENTS:

- 2 boiled sweet potatoes
- 1 tsp olive oil
- Chaat masala

DIRECTIONS:

1. Take 2 boiled sweet potatoes and cut them into roundels to make the chips.
2. Take a non-stick pan and spread 1 tsp olive oil on it.
3. Put the sweet potatoes roundels in the pan and sprinkle some chaat masala over them.
4. Cook them until they become crispy from both sides.
5. Next, transfer these chips to an air fryer to make them crispier.
6. Air fry them for about 3-5 minutes. Keep on checking them so that they don't burn.
7. Place your chips on a plate and enjoy!

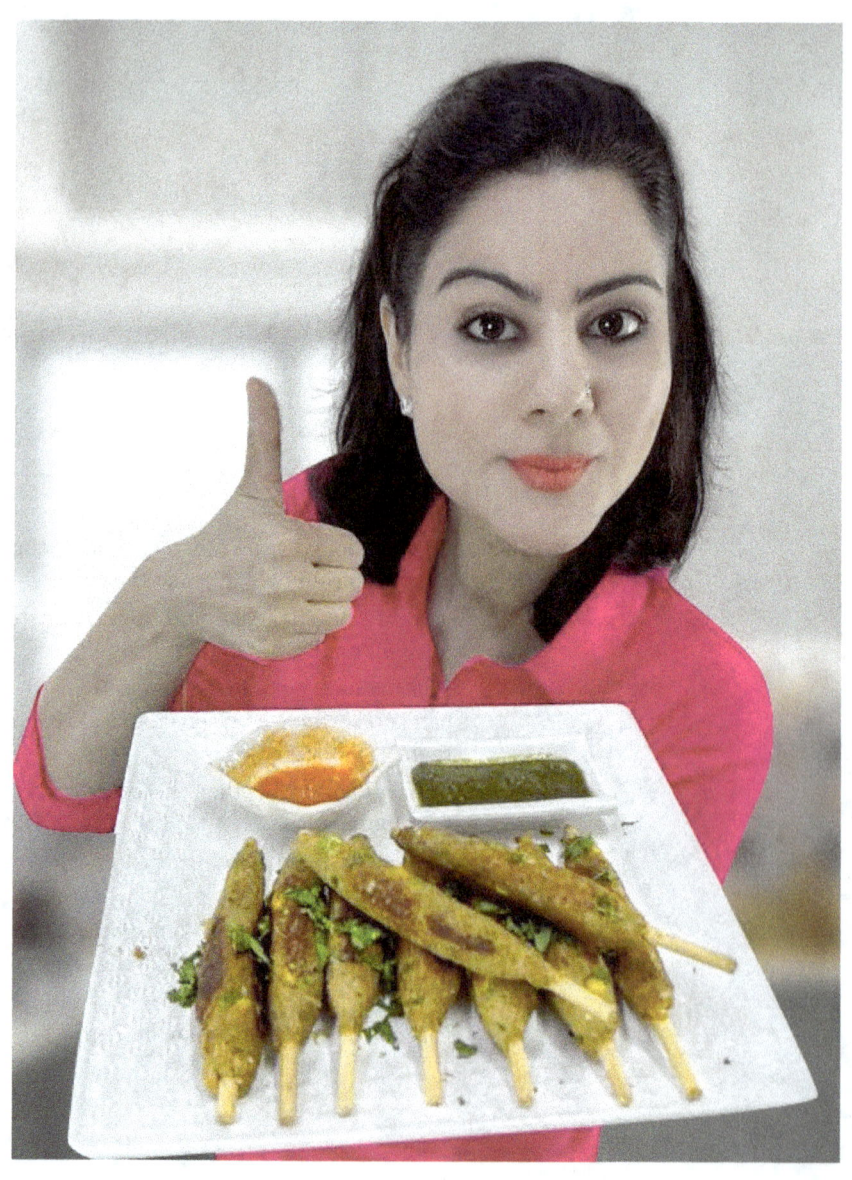

VEG KEBAB

Why should non-vegetarians have all the fun? Here's presenting the most appetizing veg kebabs recipe. Low in calories, high in nutrients! Sure, try this recipe, you'll love it! It's only 44 calories per piece of kebab!

INGREDIENTS:

- 100 grams of soya granules (soaked and squeezed)
- 8-10 coriander leaves
- 2 green chillies
- 1 tsp ginger paste
- Salt according to your taste
- 1/2 tsp cumin powder
- 1/2 tsp coriander powder
- 1/2 tsp black pepper powder
- 1/2 tsp raw mango powder
- 1 tbsp curd
- 1.5 tbsp finely chopped onions
- 1.5 tbsp boiled peas
- 1.5 tbsp grated carrots
- 1.5 tbsp boiled corns
- 1.5 tbsp beans
- 1.5 tbsp finely chopped capsicum
- 2 tbsp oats flour

DIRECTIONS:

1. In a blender, add soaked soya granules, coriander leaves, ginger, green chillies, salt, coriander powder, cumin powder, black pepper powder, and raw mango powder to it.
2. Next, add 1 tbsp curd and blend the ingredients well till they form a smooth paste.
3. Take the paste out of the blender and add onions, boiled peas, carrots, boiled corns, beans and capsicum.
4. Add oats flour to the mixture and mix all the ingredients well.
5. Take bamboo skewers and coat the kebab mixture around them properly.
6. Take a pan and spread a little oil over it and place the kebab skewers on it.
7. Cook till they are crispy from both sides.
8. Once, the kebabs are crispy put the skewers onto a plate and enjoy hot!

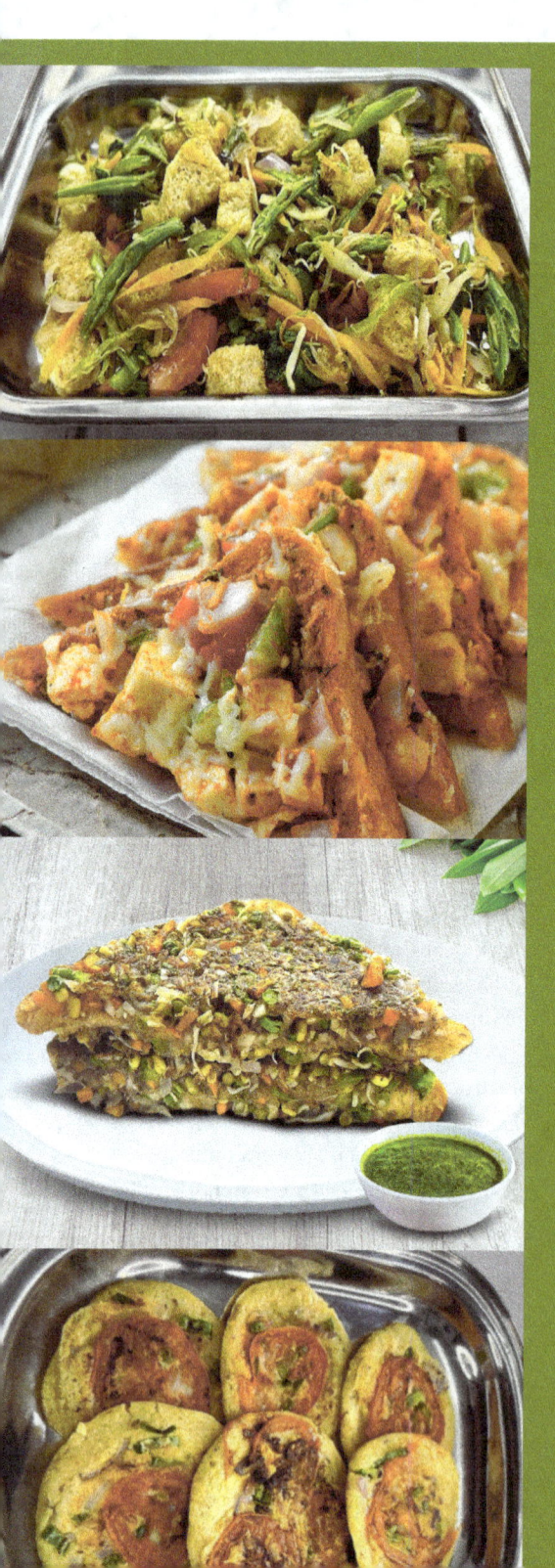

BREAKFAST

We know that every meal is vital, but breakfast is considered the most significant and crucial meal for us. It's the meal that we begin our day with. Something that keeps us energised for the whole day. You need to be very careful with what you consume during your breakfast. As if you don't start your day with something healthy and energetic, you'll end up staying lethargic the whole day. You wouldn't feel like doing anything.

There are multiple benefits of having a healthy breakfast, as it gives you the vitality to get through the whole day. It provides you with a healthy heart, boosts your metabolism and reduces the risk of diabetes and many more. Eating breakfast can also help you lose weight if consumed properly and healthily.

Many people skip their breakfast to get more sleep or get to their work on time. Or they don't know what to devour for their breakfast to lose weight. So, either they skip their breakfast or gulp something that's not healthy and leads to weight gain. But to help you free of this trouble, we have come up with delicious solutions. We have got you the best breakfast recipes that aren't only easy to make but are healthy for you too. Recipes that you can devour without the fear of being fat. We have taken care of everything! And that's why we have brought different breakfast ideas. Be it your favourite parantha, toasts, pancakes or upma. We have got you all.

These are so nourishing and quick to make that you won't even have to spend much time in the kitchen. You can comfortably make these recipes before going to work. All these recipes are quick and easy to make. You can comfortably make these with the ingredients available at home. So, now you'll never have to think about what to take for breakfast. Try these recipes and enjoy the most delicious and exciting breakfasts.

BREAD POHA

Are you tired of the same old poha recipes? Try this flavoursome bread poha recipe from Natasha Mohan. It has got all the flavours. Sure, try this as it's only 150 calories.

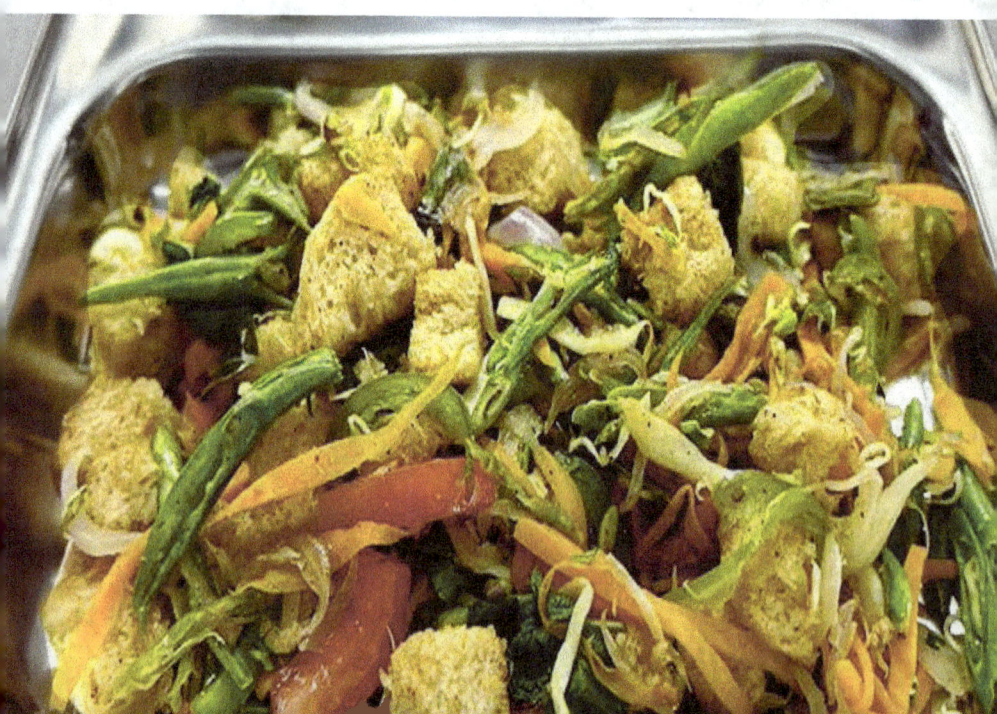

INGREDIENTS:

- 1/2 tsp oil
- 1/2 tsp mustard seeds
- 1/2 green chillies (roundels)
- 1/2 tsp curry leaves
- 1 tbsp onion (julienne)
- 1 tbsp cabbage (julienne)
- 1 tbsp carrot (julienne)
- 1 tbsp capsicum (julienne)
- 1 tbsp beans (julienne)
- Salt according to your taste
- 1/4 tsp black pepper powder
- 1/4 tsp coriander powder
- 1/4 tsp red chilli powder
- 1/4 tsp garam masala
- 1 slice of brown bread (chopped into pieces)

DIRECTIONS:

1. In a pan, add 1/2 tsp oil and let it heat for 2 minutes.

2. Now add mustard seeds, green chillies, and curry leaves. Let it sauté for 2-3 minutes until aromatic and crackling.

3. Next, add onion, carrot, capsicum, beans and cabbage. Mix the ingredients well, and sauté for 4-5 minutes on low flame.

4. Now, add salt, black pepper powder, coriander powder, red chilli powder, and garam masala. Mix spices with ingredients properly.

5. Next, take 1 slice of brown bread, chop it into pieces and add to the pan. Cook for 3-4 minutes and serve hot!

CHEESE PANEER TIKKA SANDWICH

Are you tired of the same breakfast options? Well, try this appetizing cheese paneer tikka sandwich and bring flavours to your boring breakfast routine. It's so delicious that you'll it and it's only 68 calories per slice.

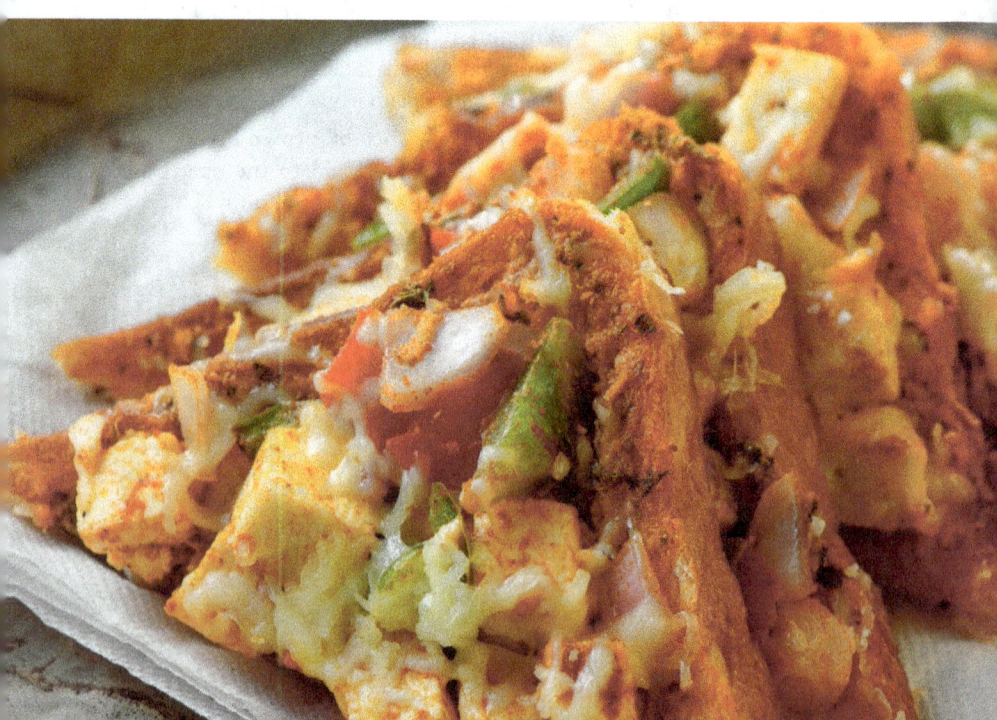

INGREDIENTS:

- 50 grams paneer (chopped into cubes)
- 1-1.5 tbsp chopped capsicum
- 1-1.5 tbsp chopped onion
- 1 tsp finely chopped coriander leaves
- 1 tbsp roasted gram flour (besan)
- 1 tbsp hung curd
- Salt according to your taste
- 1/2 tsp garam masala
- 1 tsp coriander powder
- 1/2 tsp red chilli powder
- 1/2 tsp mustard oil
- 4 atta bread slices
- green chutney
- 1 tsp cheddar cheese
- 1/2 tsp oil

INGREDIENTS:

- Chilli flakes
- Oregano

DIRECTIONS:

1. Take a bowl and add paneer cubes, capsicum, onion, chopped coriander leaves, gram flour and hung curd.

2. Next, add garam masala, coriander powder, salt, red chilli powder and 1/2 tsp mustard oil.

3. Now, mix all the ingredients well until the paneer and vegetables are coated properly.

4. Take 2 atta bread slices and chop the centre part of one bread, keep the edges only. While keeping the other one as it is. Repeat the same process with the other 2.

5. Apply green chutney over the bread pieces and take the edges of the bread and put them over it.

6. Now, put the paneer stuffing in the empty space between and sprinkle cheddar cheese over it.

7. Take a non-stick pan and spread 1/2 tsp oil over it properly. Now, take your paneer sandwich and put it in the pan. Cover the pan with a lid.

8. After 3 minutes, flip your bread over and cook until crispy from both sides.

9. Transfer the paneer tikka cheese sandwich to a plate and garnish it with some chilli flakes and oregano. Enjoy!

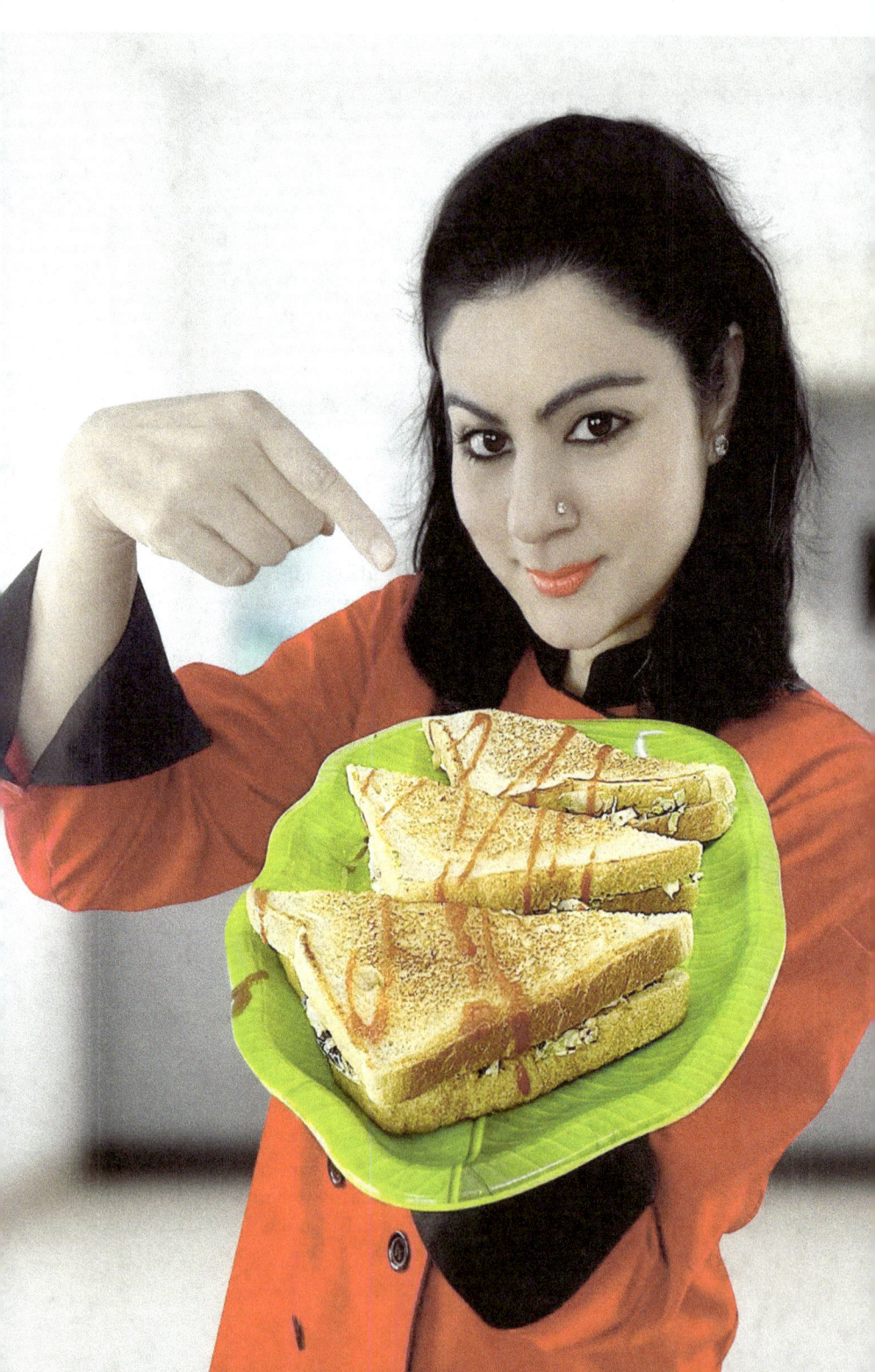

EGG SANDWICH*

Some crispy, healthy, filling and mouth-watering egg sandwiches for breakfast. Loaded with protein and so easy to make. Only 90 calories per slice. Sure, try this once and you'll want to relish it daily.

INGREDIENTS:

- 1 tbsp finely chopped onion
- 1 tbsp finely chopped carrot
- 1 tbsp finely chopped capsicum
- 1 tbsp finely chopped/ grated cabbage
- 1 tsp finely chopped coriander leaves
- 1 tsp olives
- 1/2 tsp chilli flakes
- 1 Salt according to your taste
- 1/2 tsp oregano
- 1/2 tsp black pepper powder
- 2 tbsp hung curd
- 1 tsp mustard sauce
- 2 boiled and finely chopped egg whites (no yellow)
- 2 whole wheat slices of bread

DIRECTIONS:

1. For the filling, take a bowl and add finely chopped onion, carrot, capsicum and cabbage.
2. Now add chopped coriander leaves and olives to it.
3. Next, add chilli flakes, salt, oregano, black pepper powder and hung curd.
4. Now add mustard sauce and mix all the ingredients well.
5. Now boil 2 eggs and only take egg whites. Remove egg yellow from it and finely chop the egg whites.
6. Then, take these finely chopped egg whites and transfer them to the filling bowl.
7. Now take 2 slices of bread and spread half the filling over any one of them. Put another bread over it.
8. Next, take a pan and apply a little oil to it and put the bread over it. Cook until the bread gets brown and crispy from both sides.
9. Transfer the egg sandwich to the plate. Cut it in half and enjoy!

NOTES:

Contain egg

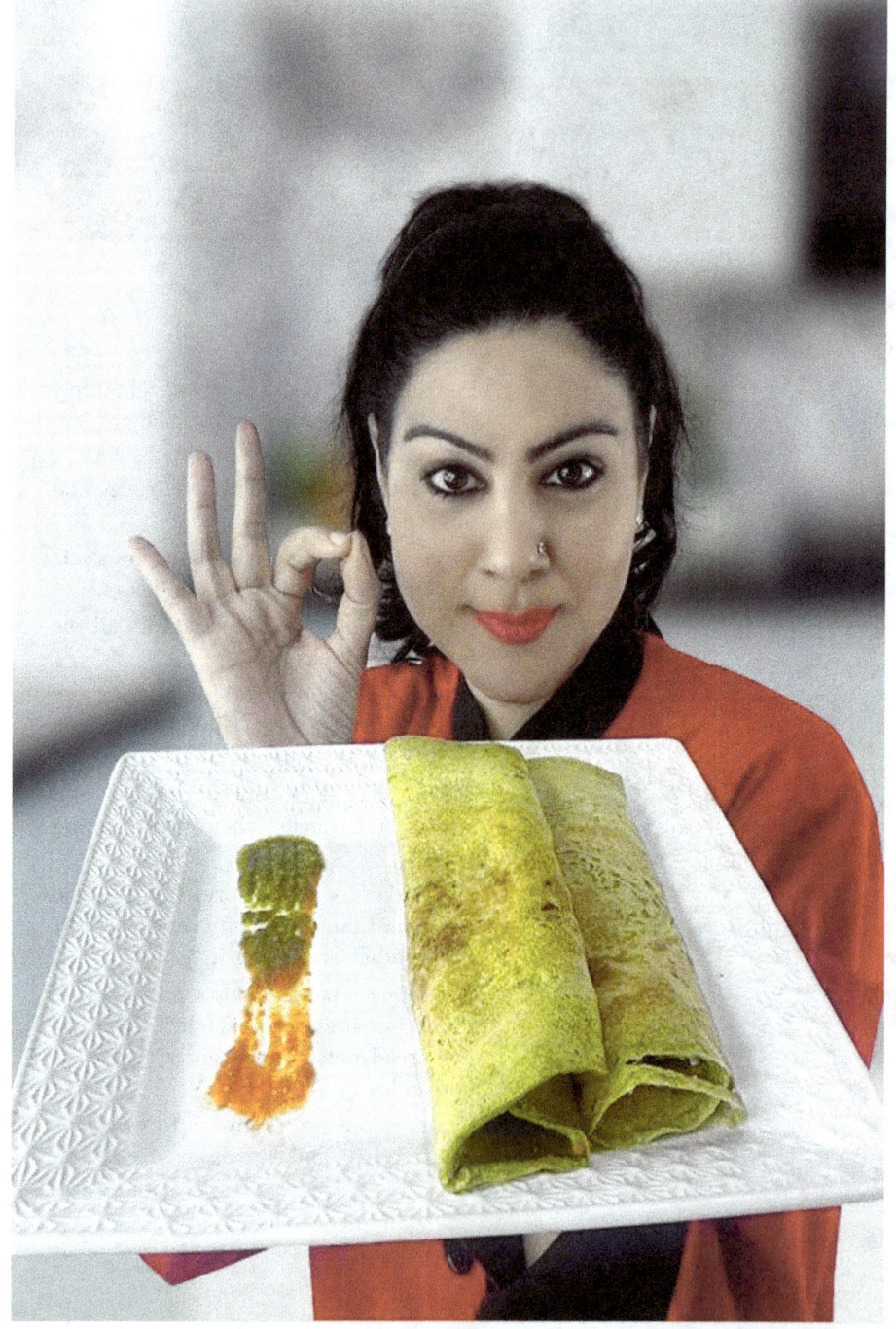

MOONG DAL CHEELA

Looking for some quick breakfast options? Try this quick and easy-to-make moong dal cheela recipe. You'll love it! It's loaded with flavours and the best part is, it's only 120 calories per cheela.

INGREDIENTS:

- 100 grams soaked moong dal (green)
- 6-7 curry leaves
- Salt according to your taste
- 2 green chillies
- 1/2 inch ginger
- 1/2 tsp cumin seeds Water
- 1/2 tsp finely chopped onion
- 1/2 tsp finely chopped tomato
- 1/2 tsp finely chopped paneer
- Pinch of black pepper powder
- 1/2 tsp finely chopped coriander leaves

DIRECTIONS:

1. In a blender, add soaked moong dal, curry leaves, salt, green chillies, ginger, cumin seeds and water. Blend until smooth.

2. Take a pan and brush it with a little oil. Then pour some batter over the pan and let it cook on low flame for 2-3 minutes.

3. Add chopped onions, tomatoes, paneer, a pinch of black pepper, a pinch of salt and coriander leaves.

4. Let it cook for 1-2 minutes. Fold the cheela and transfer it to a plate and enjoy!

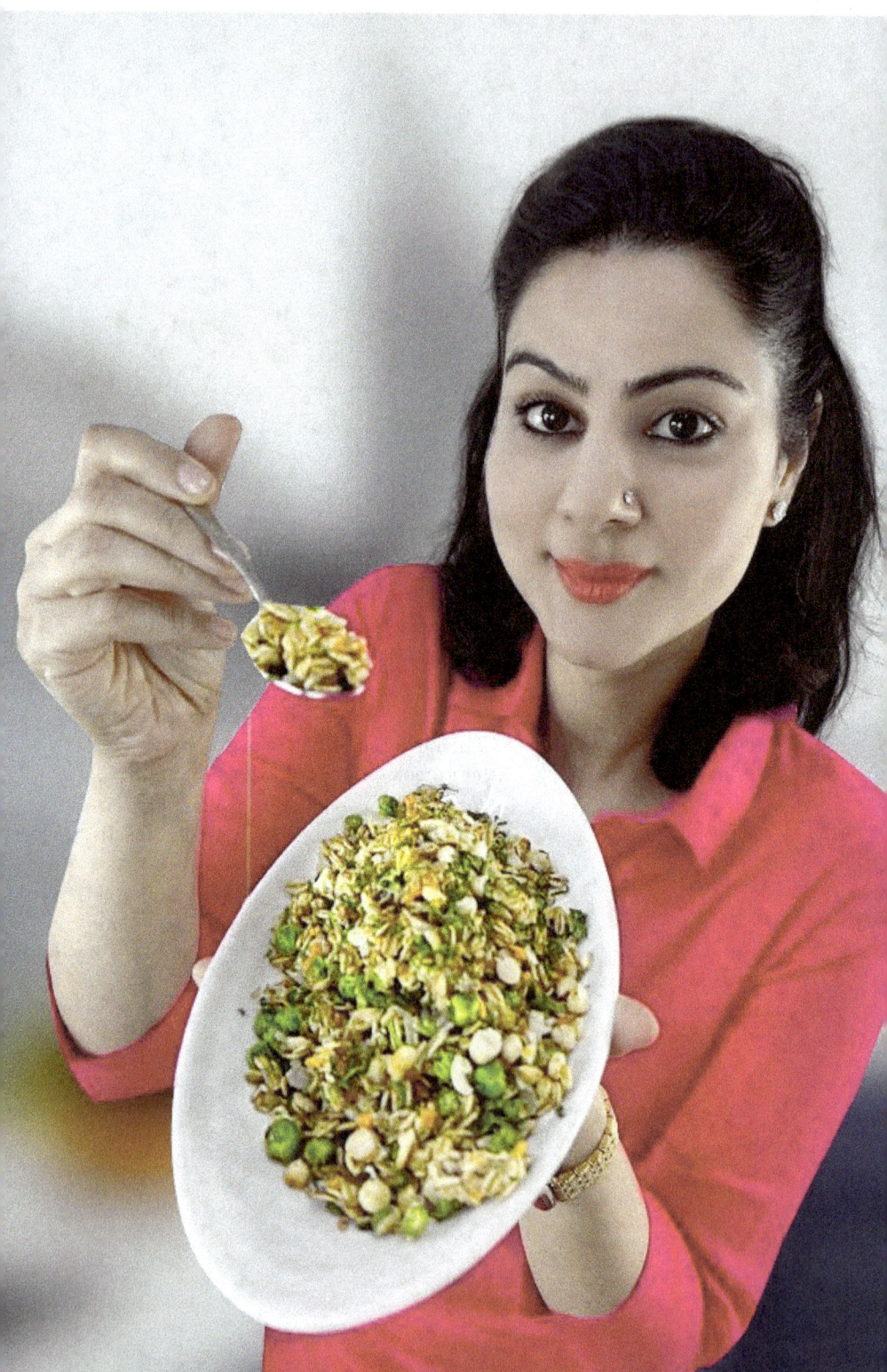

OATS & EGG UPMA*

Looking for a protein-rich breakfast? We have got one! Try this mouth-watering 198 calories oats and egg upma recipe, it will fulfil all your protein requirements that too within limited calories.

INGREDIENTS:

- 1/2 tsp oil
- 1/2 tsp mustard seeds
- 1 tsp green chillies (fine roundels)
- 1.5 tbsp finely chopped onion.
- 1 tbsp finely chopped beans
- 1 tbsp finely chopped carrot
- 1 tbsp boiled peas
- 30 grams rolled oats
- Salt according to your taste
- 1/2 tsp Black pepper powder
- 1 tsp finely chopped coriander leaves
- 2 egg whites (no yellow part)

DIRECTIONS:

1. In a frying pan add 1/2 tsp oil, mustard seeds, green chillies, and onion. Sauté the onions on a low flame for 2-3 minutes until they turn golden brown.

2. Now add beans, carrots, boiled peas, and rolled oats. Let it cook for 3-4 minutes on a low flame.

3. Next, add salt and black pepper powder. Mix all the ingredients well and let it cook until the colour of the oats changes to light brown.

4. Now add chopped coriander leaves and egg whites. Cook for another 2-3 minutes.

5. Transfer the egg upma to a plate and garnish with roasted peanut and, enjoy!

Note:

Contain egg

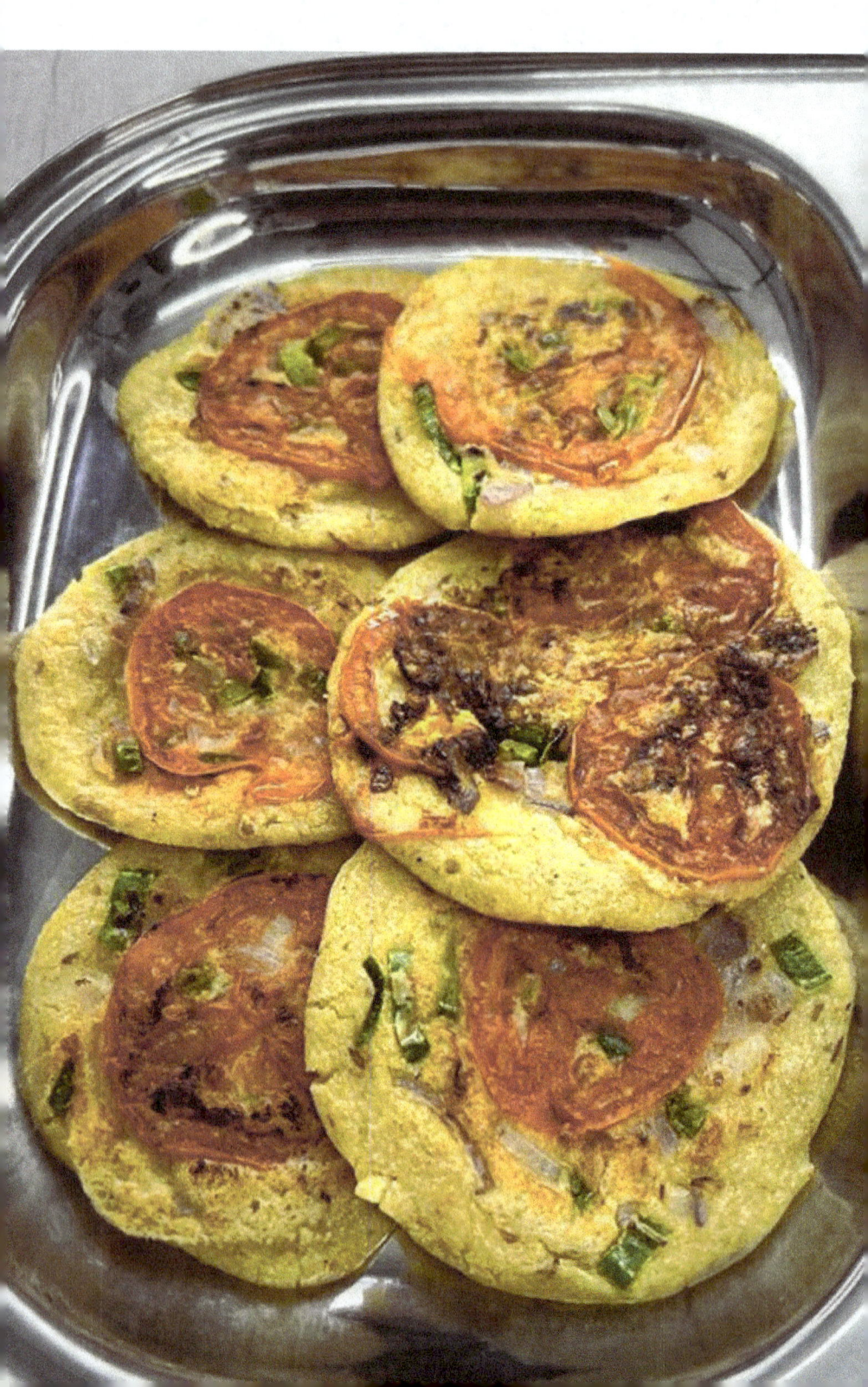

OATS & MOONG DAL PANCAKE

Don't like oats? No, problem! But you'll like it this way! Try these delectable oats and moong dal pancakes and we assure you, you will fall in love with oats.

Perfect for your child's tiffin as well as yours! It's 44 calories per piece of pancake.

INGREDIENTS:

- 50 grams moong dal
- 50 grams oats
- 1/4 tsp fenugreek seeds
- 1/2 tsp cumin seeds
- 1/4 tsp asafoetida (hing)
- Salt according to your taste
- 1/4 tsp garam masala
- 1/2 tsp coriander powder
- 2-3 small paneer cubes
- 1 tbsp finely chopped onion
- 1 tbsp finely chopped capsicum
- 1 tomato (chopped into thin roundels)

DIRECTIONS:

1. In a bowl, add moong dal, oats, fenugreek seeds, and cumin seeds. Add water and soak the mixture for about 1/2 hour. Cover it and keep it aside.

2. Now, after 1/2 hour, pour the soaked mixture into the blender and add salt, asafoetida, coriander powder, and garam masala to it. Blend the mixture into a smooth paste.

3. Take a non-stick pan and spread the mixture over it. Give it a small pancake shape.

4. Decorate it with onions, capsicum, paneer and tomato.

5. Flip the oats and moong dal pancakes to another side carefully. Cook from both sides and enjoy!

PIZZA SANDWICH

Who says you can't have your favourite pizza in your weight loss journey? Of course, you can have it, but with my healthy twist! Just like my pizza sandwich!

Loaded with vegetables and so delicious! It only contains 183 calories!

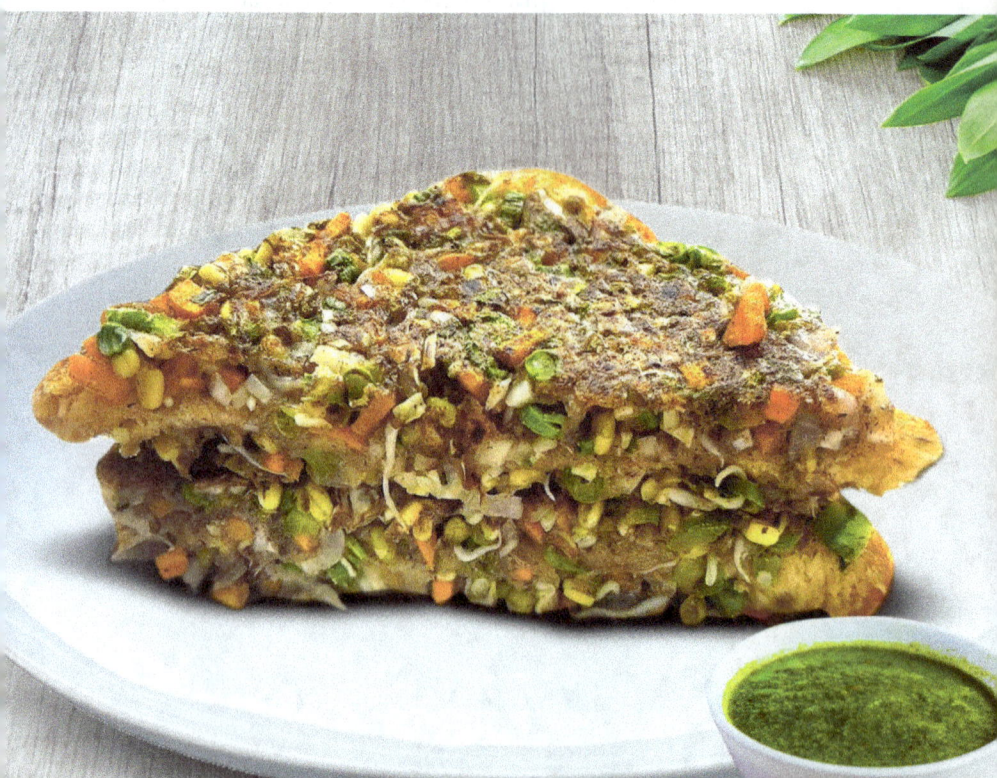

INGREDIENTS:

- 1.5 tbsp ragi flour
- Salt according to your taste
- 1/4 tsp cumin powder
- 1/2 tsp raw mango powder (amchur)
- 1/4 tsp black pepper powder
- 1/4 tsp carom seeds
- 6-7 tbsp water
- 1 tsp chopped coriander leaves
- 1 tbsp finely chopped onion
- 1 tbsp finely chopped capsicum
- 1 tbsp finely chopped beans
- 1 tbsp finely chopped carrot
- 30 grams sprouts
- 1 tbsp finely chopped cabbage
- 1/2 tsp ghee
- 1 atta bread

DIRECTIONS:

1. In a bowl add ragi flour, salt, cumin powder, raw mango powder, black pepper powder, carom seeds, and 5-6 tbsp water. Mix it well until it forms a paste.

2. Now, add chopped coriander, onion, capsicum, beans, carrot, sprouts, and cabbage.

3. Next, add 1-2 spoons of water and mix all the ingredients well. (Add water as required)

4. Take a non-stick pan and apply 1/2 tsp oil to it. Spread it over the pan.

5. Next, take an atta bread and put it in the pan. Once it gets crispy from one side, flip it over to another and apply our pizza filling to it. Spread the filling properly.

6. Now, after the other side gets crispy, flip the bread carefully and let the pizza filling cook.

7. Now, spread the rest pizza filling to the empty side of the bread and flip the bread again carefully. Cook until the filling is done. (You can use ghee, so the filling doesn't stick with the pan.)

8. Take the pizza sandwich out of the pan and transfer it to a plate. Cut it from between and enjoy!

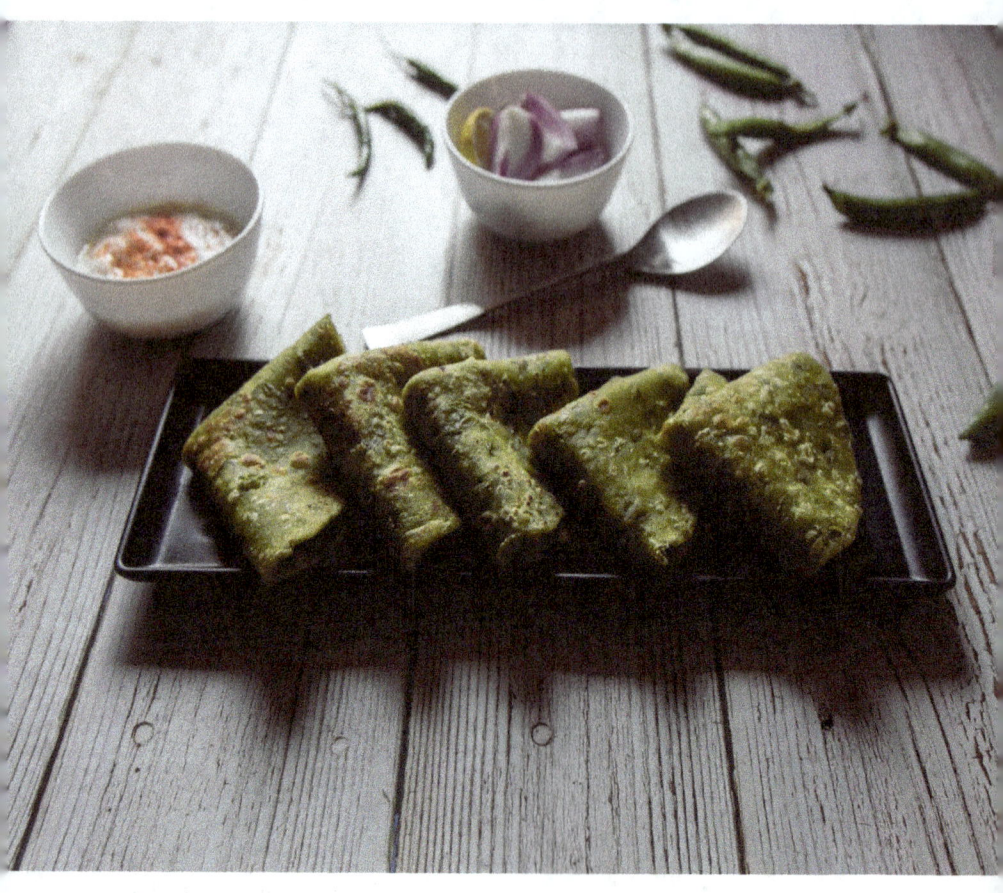

SPROUTS STUFFED PARANTHA

For all those who can't get enough of paranthas. It's not an ordinary parantha, it's stuffed with the goodness of sprouts and only contains 183 calories. It's so healthy and filling that you won't feel hungry for long. It will provide you with the energy to get throughout the day!

INGREDIENTS:

- 50 grams sprouts (raw)
- 2-3 black pepper corn kernels (raw)
- 1/4 tsp carom seeds (ajwain)
- 1/4 tsp cumin seeds
- 1/4 tsp fennel seeds
- 1 small-sized green chilli
- 1/2 inch ginger
- 1 tbsp boiled peas
- 1 tbsp finely chopped onion
- 1 tsp chopped coriander leaves
- Salt according to your taste
- A pinch of garam masala
- 1/2 tsp raw mango powder (amchur)
- 1/4 tsp coriander powder
- A pinch of red chilli powder
- 1/2 tsp ghee

For roti:

- Whole wheat flour
- Water

DIRECTIONS:

1. Take a blender and add sprouts, black pepper corn kernels, carom seeds, cumin seeds, fennel seeds, green chilli, and ginger to it. Blend the mixture properly.

2. Transfer the blended mixture to a bowl and add boiled peas, onion, and coriander leaves to it.

3. Now add salt, garam masala, raw mango powder, coriander powder, and red chilli powder. Mix all the ingredients well.

4. Next, take whole wheat flour and add water to it. Knead the dough like you usually knead your roti dough.

5. Roll 2 thin rotis. Take one rolled roti and spread the sprout mixture over it. Cover it with another roti and roll it properly.

6. Now take a non-stick pan and carefully pick up the parantha and put it in the pan.

7. Spread ghee over parantha and flip it to another side. Cook until it gets crispy.

8. Serve hot and enjoy!

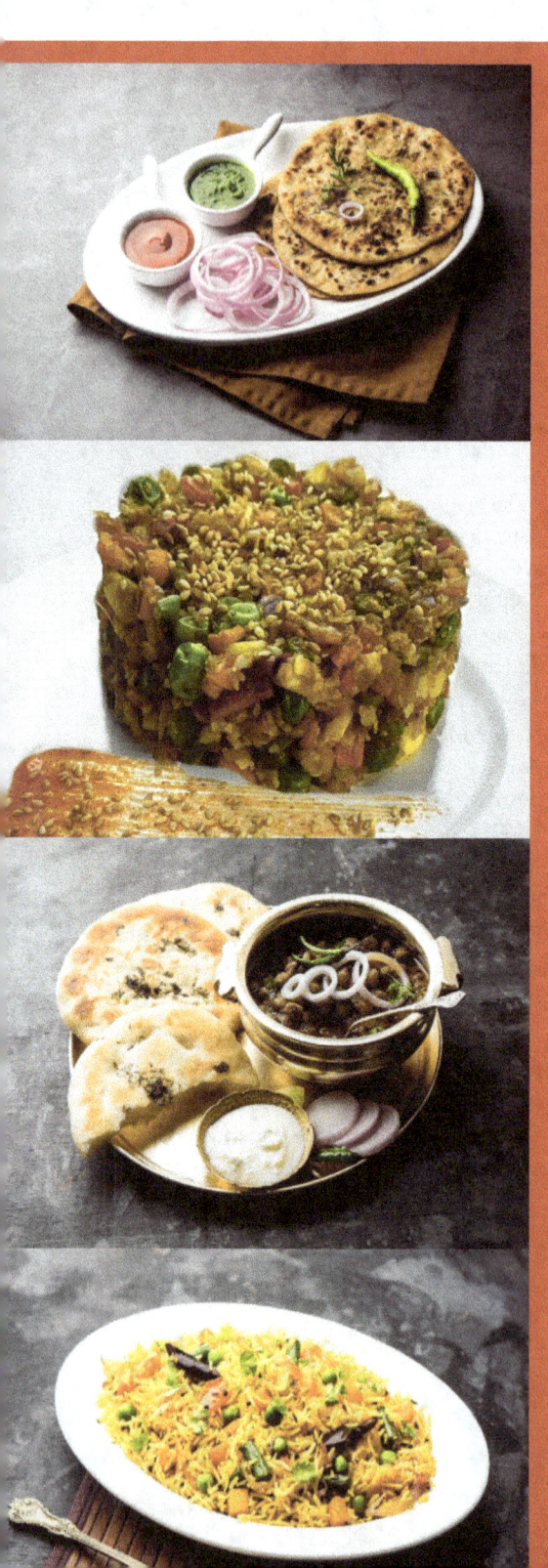

LUNCH

When we talk about weight loss, there are a lot of things that come to our minds. Like eating a protein-rich diet, intermittent fasting, and eating less and often. But what if it was simple when it comes to eating or losing weight? There's no such thing as eating less to lose weight. Instead, eating balanced meals to lose weight always works.

Most people just skip their mid-nay meals or lunch to lose weight. But they don't know that this doesn't help in losing weight instead, they end up eating more calories. Those who skip their lunches often feel hungry and eat whatever comes in front of them. This leads to eating more and consuming more calories than usual. So why not eat your lunches?

We know that consuming a healthy lunch is not always possible, especially when you're busy with your work or family. The idea of making a separate meal that is healthy enough to lose weight is always a buzzkill. That's why to avoid this situation and to help you out. We have brought you lunch recipes that are healthy and scrumptious at the same time. And the best part is you don't have to cook something special for yourself to lose weight. You can eat what your family eats. As these recipes are so delicious that everyone loves to relish them. Even your kids will love these recipes. These recipes are for all your needs, be it a weight loss parantha, tangy chaat papdi, fried rice, salads, or desi kulchey choley. We have all!

We know you must be thinking that these will take a lot of time to get cooked but no! These are timesaving, quick and easy-to-make recipes that anyone can make. So, with our recipes, you wouldn't have to skip your lunches anymore. You can now comfortably relish them without thinking about your weight. As these recipes help in weight loss too!

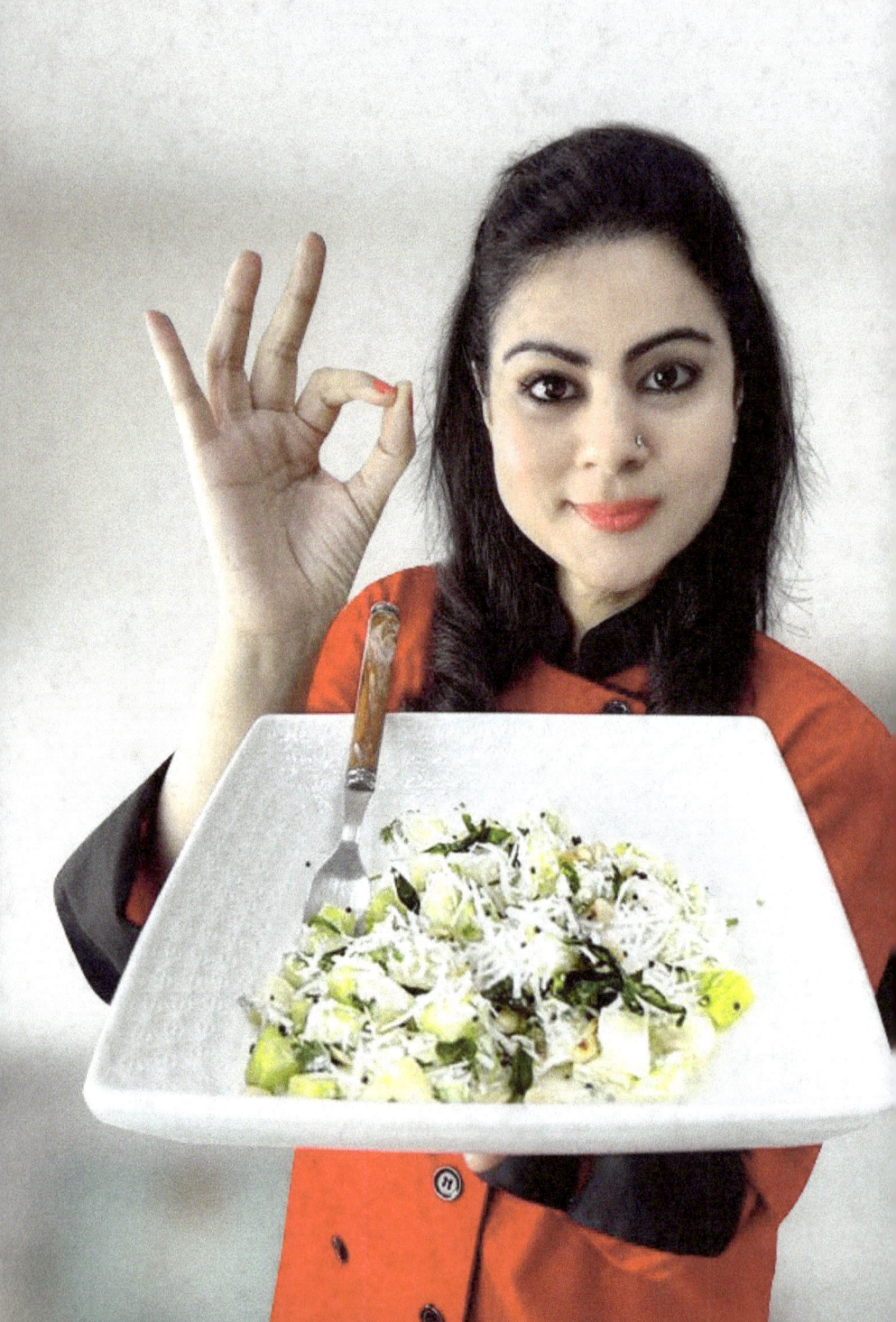

CUCUMBER COCONUT SALAD

For all those who want to relish something unique and refreshing for lunch. Try this amazing cucumber coconut salad recipe and feel the difference. And it's only 163 calories! You'll love it!

INGREDIENTS:

- 1 cucumber chopped
- 1 tbsp chopped coriander leaves
- 1 tsp green chilli roundels
- 1 tbsp hung curd
- 1 tsp mustard seeds
- 1 tbsp curry leaves
- 1 tbsp peanuts
- 2 tbsp grated coconut

DIRECTIONS:

1. Take a plate and add cucumber pieces, chopped coriander leaves, green chilli roundels and hung curd. Mix all the ingredients well.

2. For tempering, take a non-stick pan and add 1 tsp of oil to it. Then, add mustard seeds, curry leaves, and peanuts. Cook until mustard seeds start to crackle.

3. Now add grated coconut over the cucumber and hung curd mixture.

4. Now, pour the tempering over the plate and voila your cucumber coconut salad is ready. Enjoy!

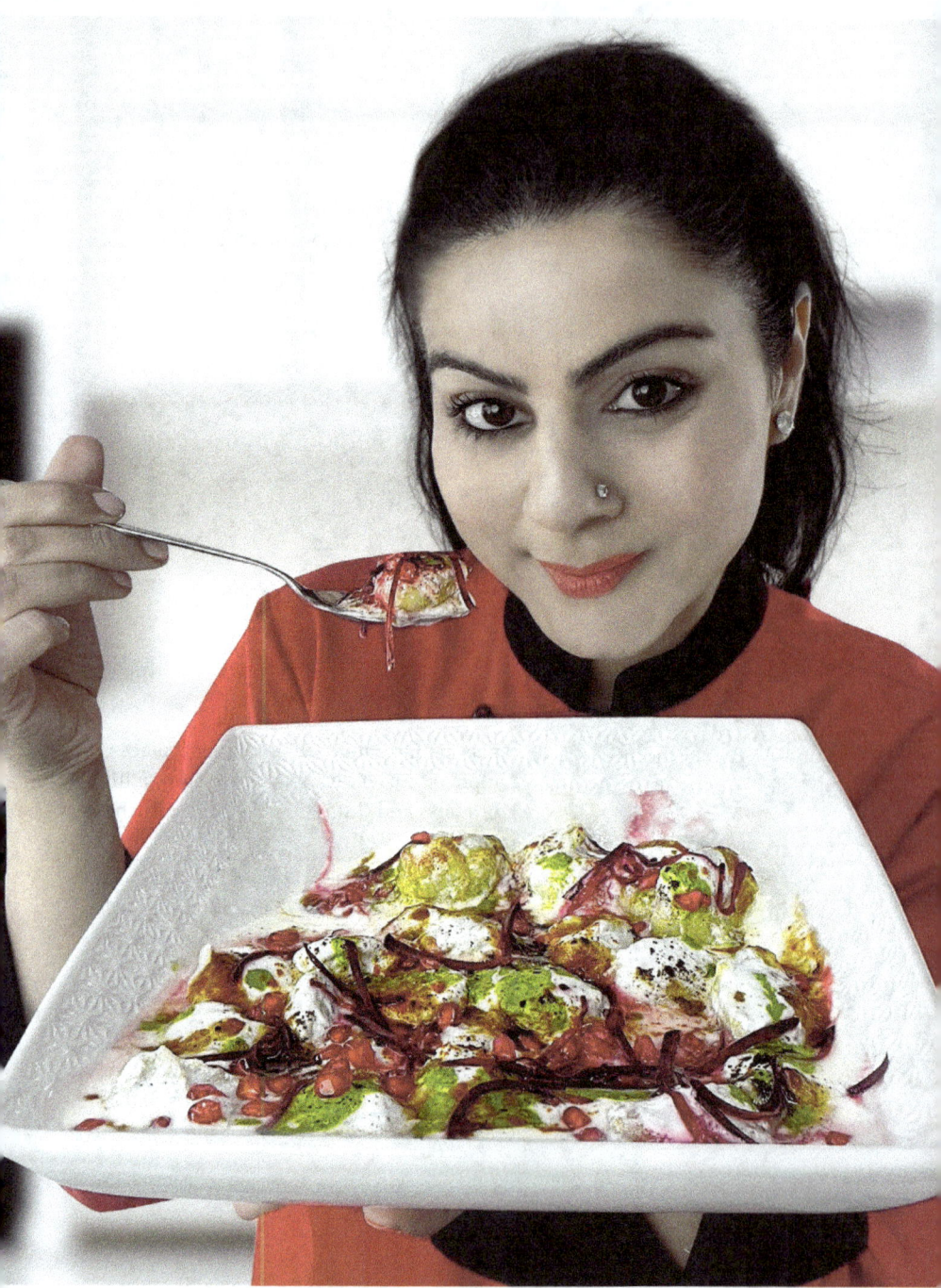

Note:

Use a toothpick to check if the dhokla is cooked or not. Take the toothpick, put it in the dhokla, and check if it's clear or not. If it's clear, then the dhokla Is cooked. Otherwise, let it cook for more minutes.

DAHI BHALLA

Have you ever heard of no-oil Dahi Bhalla? Well, if you haven't, try these 20 calories per piece dahi bhalla recipe! It's best when you want to relish something different and quick.

INGREDIENTS:

- 50 grams urad dal (soaked overnight)
- 150 grams moong chilka dal (soaked overnight)
- 1/2 inch ginger
- 2 green chillies
- Salt according to your taste
- Oil (to grease the mould)
- Hot water
- A pinch asafoetida (hing)
- 1 cup beaten curd
- 1 tsp homemade dates chutney
- 1 tsp homemade green chutney
- 1/2 tsp red chilli powder
- 1/2 tsp chaat masala
- 1/2 tsp black salt

Garnish

- Pomegranate seeds
- Thinly sliced beetroot juliennes

DIRECTIONS:

1. In a bowl add 50 grams urad dal, 150 grams moong chilka dal and water. Wash the dal 2 times and soak them overnight.

2. Next, take a blender and add soaked urad dal, soaked moong chilka dal, ginger, green chillies, and salt. Blend until a smooth paste is formed.

3. Transfer the mixture into a bowl. Using a hand blender, blend it until fluffy.

4. Take an idli steamer, grease it with a little oil and transfer this batter to it using a tsp.

5. Steam it for about 5-7 minutes on a low flame until cooked.

6. Now, take a bowl and pour hot water into it. Transfer the bhallas into the bowl and add a pinch of asafoetida to it. Let the bhallas soak in the water for 5-7 minutes.

7. After 5-7 minutes, squeeze the bhallas properly and transfer them to a plate.

8. Take 1 bowl of curd and beat it properly until it gets smooth. Spread the beaten curd all over the bhallas.

9. Next, add homemade dates chutney and green chutney to it. Sprinkle some red chilli powder, chaat masala, and black salt.

10. Garnish it with pomegranate seeds and thin beetroot juliennes and enjoy your no-oil dahi bhalla!

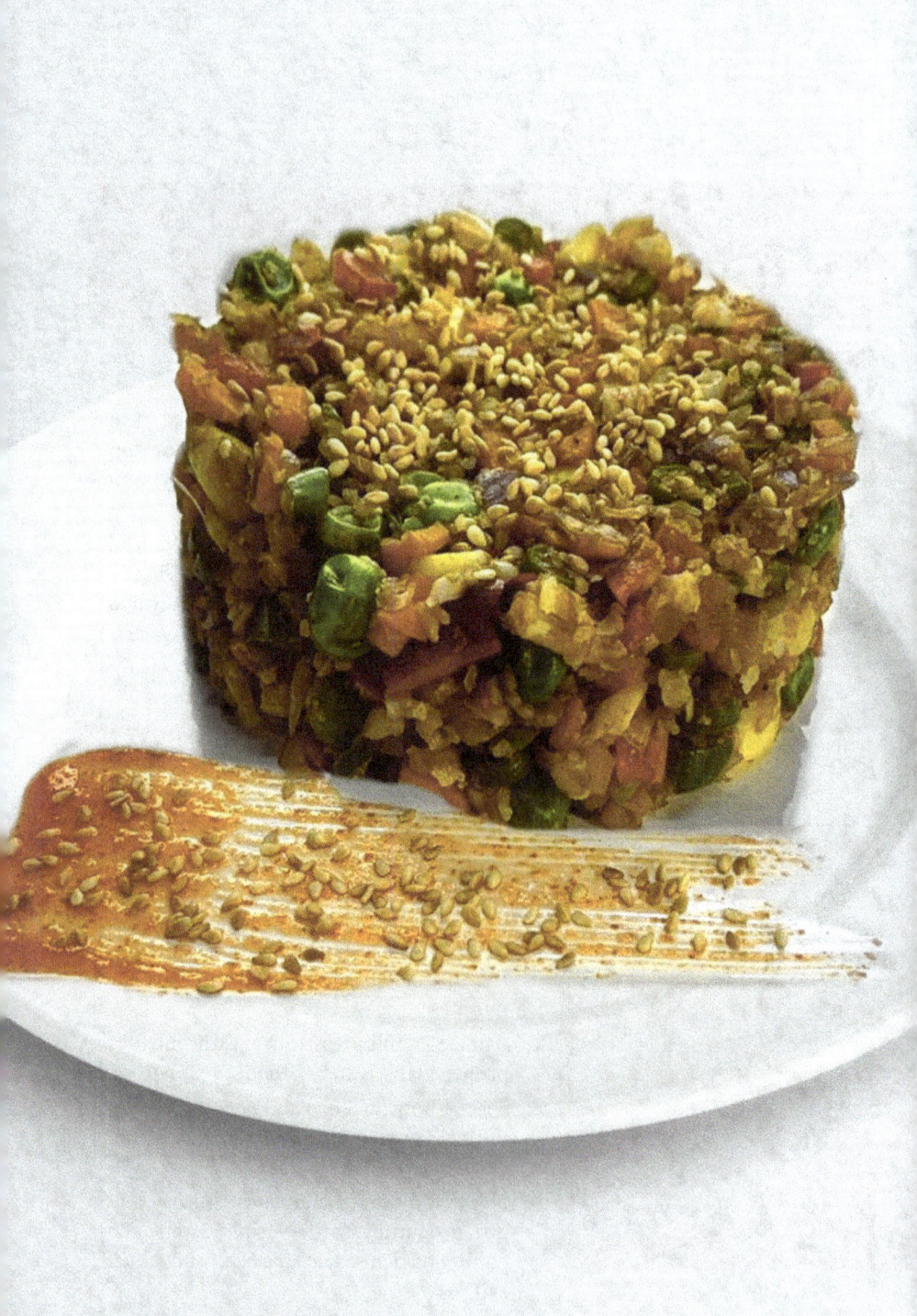

FRIED RICE

Who says dieting is boring? Try this flavoursome, 136 calories fried rice recipe.

Once you try this, you will fall in love! It's loaded with the goodness of vegetables. You can add your preferred vegetable and enjoy this.

INGREDIENTS:

- 1.5 tsp sesame oil
- 2 dried red chillies
- (torn and de-seeded)
- 1/2 tsp chopped ginger
- 1-1.5 tsp minced garlic
- 40 grams chopped onions
- 40 grams chopped carrots
- 40 grams of chopped beans
- 200 grams grated cauliflower
- 40 grams boiled peas
- 3 tbsp chopped bell peppers (red, green and yellow)
- 1 tsp soy sauce
- 1 tsp vinegar
- 1 tsp black pepper powder
- Salt according to your taste

DIRECTIONS:

1. In a wok, add 1.5 tsp sesame oil, dried red chillies, ginger, and garlic to it. Sauté it for 2-3 minutes on a low flame until turns golden.

2. Next, add chopped onions, carrots, and beans. Mix well and sauté for 2-3 minutes.

3. Now, add grated cauliflower to it. Cover it and cook it for 5 minutes on a low flame.

4. After 5 minutes, add boiled peas, boiled corns, and chopped bell peppers.

5. Now, add soy sauce, vinegar, black pepper powder, and salt. Mix all the ingredients well. Cook for 2 minutes. Serve hot and enjoy!

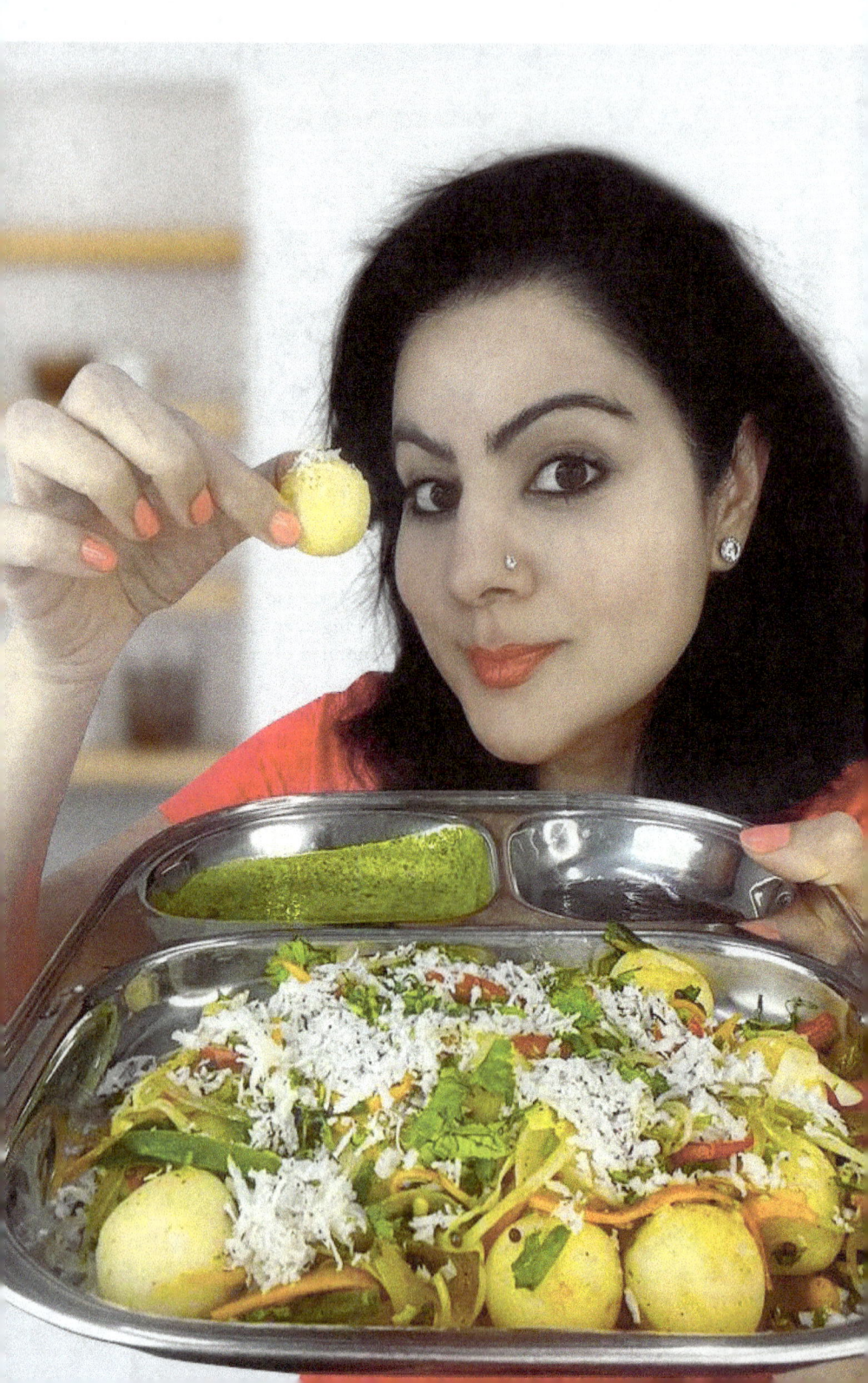

GOLI IDLI

It's time for some goli idlis! A perfect meal option for those who don't want to have something heavy. Quick and easy-to-make option! Only 25 calories per goli idli!

INGREDIENTS:

- 1 cup water
- 100 grams rice flour
- Salt according to your taste
- 1/2 tsp chilli flakes
- 1 tsp oil
- 1 tbsp mustard seeds
- 1 green chilli (roundels)
- 7-8 curry leaves
- 1/2 tsp urad dal
- 1/2 tsp chana dal
- 2 tbsp onions
- 2 tbsp capsicum
- 2 tbsp carrot
- 2 tbsp cabbage
- Salt according to your taste
- 1/2 tsp black pepper powder
- Chopped coriander leaves

GARNISH:

- Grated coconut

DIRECTIONS:

1. In a frying pan, add 1 cup of water and rice flour.
2. Next, add salt and chilli flakes. Cook it on low flame till it cooks properly. It will make it in dough-paste form.
3. Transfer the paste into a bowl and let it get cool. After it's cooled, we'll take a tsp with its help to make all the balls of the same size. Use your hand to give them a round ball shape.
4. Steam the idlis for about 5-7 minutes.
5. Next, take a frying pan and add 1 tsp oil, 1 tbsp mustard seeds, chopped green chillies, curry leaves, urad dal, and chana dal.
6. Now, add thinly sliced onions, capsicum, carrot, and cabbage.
7. Sauté the vegetables for 3-5 minutes. Then, add salt, black pepper, and a lot of chopped coriander leaves. Mix the ingredients well.
8. Now, add the goli idlis and sauté properly.
9. Transfer the goli idlis to a plate and sprinkle some grated coconut over the goli idlis and enjoy!

KULCHEY CHOLEY

Want to devour something exciting? Try this appetizing 141 calories kulchey choley recipe made with little oil. Who says you can't enjoy street food during your diet? With our recipes, you can!

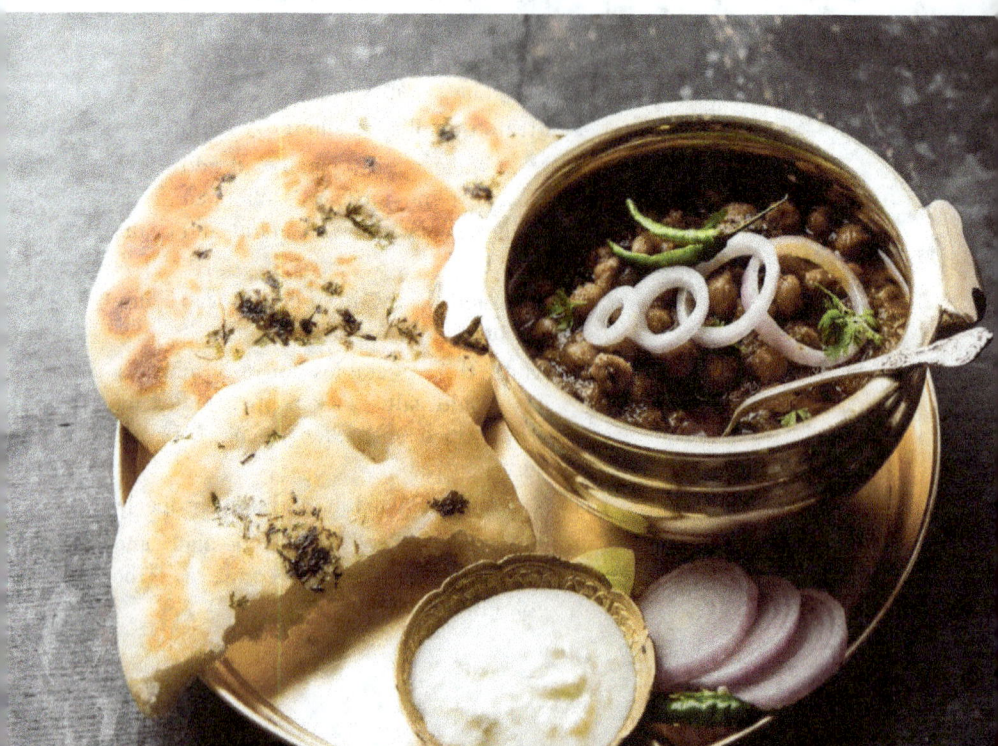

INGREDIENTS:

- 2 tbsp oil
- 1 tsp cumin seeds
- 1 tbsp thinly sliced ginger julienne
- 1 tbsp pomegranate seeds (anardana)
- 3-4 green chillies (chopped from between)
- Approximately 2 tbsp chana masala
- 1 tsp red chilli powder
- 1 tsp raw mango powder (amchur)
- Salt according to your taste
- A bowl of boiled chickpeas
- Whole wheat kulchey

GARNISH:

- Coriander leaves

DIRECTIONS:

1. In a frying pan add oil, and cumin seeds and roast them for 1-2 minutes.

2. Now add ginger slices and sauté for 3-4 minutes until aromatic.

3. Next, add pomegranate seeds, and green chillies to it. Mix well and add a little water so that the spices don't burn.

4. Now add chana masala, red chilli powder, raw mango powder, and salt. Mix all the spices well and add a little water to them. Mix it well.

5. Next, add boiled chickpeas and cook for 5-10 minutes on a high flame.

6. Turn off the heat and transfer your chana masala to a bowl. Garnish with some fresh coriander leaves.

7. Next, take whole wheat kulchey and cook them on a non-stick pan without adding any oil, and enjoy!

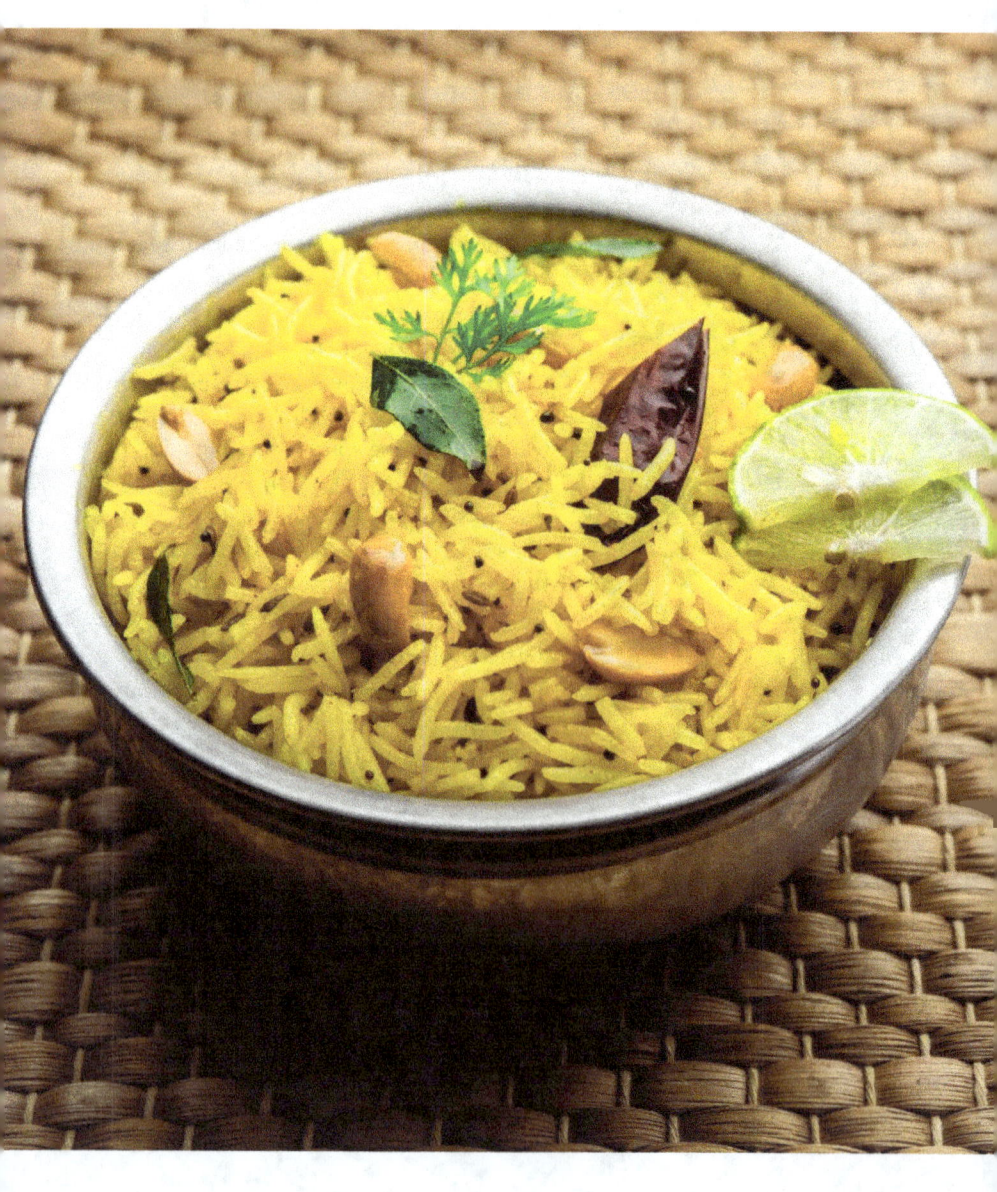

LEMON RICE

For all the rice admirers, here is a recipe that you must try! This lemon rice recipe is so good that you'll want to eat it again and again. And the best part is that it's only 221 calories!

INGREDIENTS:

- 1 tsp oil
- 1 tsp mustard seeds
- 1/4 tsp urad dal
- 1/4 tsp chana dal
- 2 whole red chillies
- 1 tsp chopped ginger
- 1 tsp green chillies (roundels)
- 1 tbsp chopped curry leaves
- 1 tsp turmeric powder
- 100 grams boiled rice
- Salt according to your taste
- 1/4 tsp garam masala
- 3/4 bowl curd (made with skimmed milk)
- Half lemon
- 1/2 tsp peanuts

DIRECTIONS:

1. Take a wok and add 1 tsp of oil to it. Heat it for 2- 3 minutes.

2. Then, add mustard seeds, urad dal, and chana dal to it. Cook until it crackles and gets aromatic on a low flame.

3. Next, add whole red chillies, ginger, green chillies, and curry leaves. Sauté for 1-2 minutes on a low flame.

4. Now add turmeric powder, boiled rice, salt, and garam masala. Mix with light hands.

5. Next, add curd, peanuts and lemon juice. Give it a nice mix and voilà your lemon rice is ready, Enjoy!

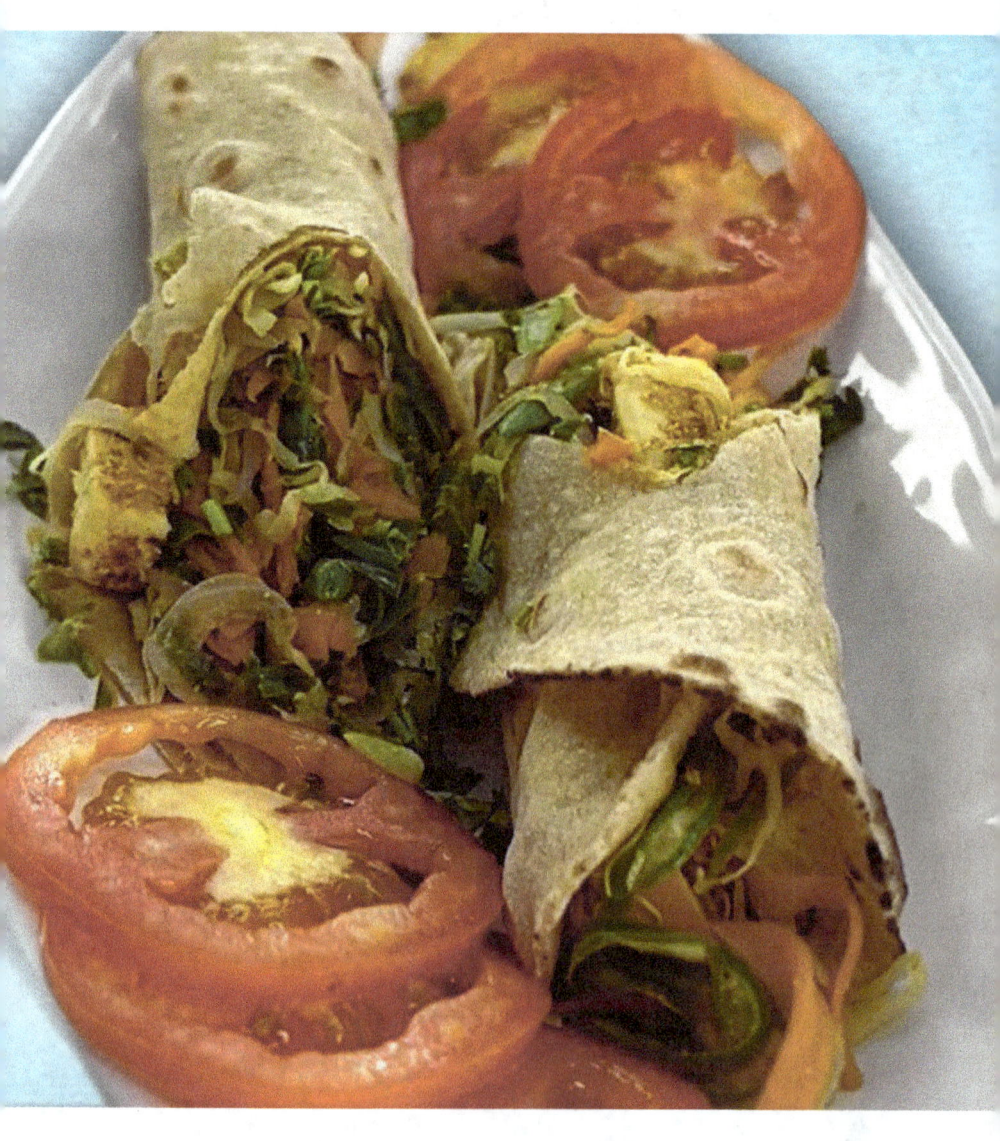

PANEER ROLL

Everyone loves Kathi roll but it contains too much oil. So, why not try this wholesome, 165 calories Kathi roll recipe? It contains so much less oil and is very healthy. Those who don't like vegetables can also relish vegetables with this recipe.

INGREDIENTS:

- 1/2 tsp oil
- 1 tbsp thinly sliced onion
- 1 tbsp thinly sliced cabbage
- 1 tbsp thinly sliced carrot
- 1 chopped green chilli
- 1 tbsp chopped beans
- 30 grams paneer chopped into cubes
- 1 tbsp curd
- 10 grams chaat masala
- 1/4 tsp garlic paste
- 1 tsp lemon juice
- 1/4 tsp red chilli powder
- 1/4 tsp coriander powder
- 1 tsp chopped coriander leaves
- 1 wheat roti
- 1 tsp homemade green chutney

DIRECTIONS:

1. Take a non-stick pan and add 1/2 tsp oil. Then add onion, cabbage, green chilli, and beans. Sauté the vegetables for 2-3 minutes on low flame.

2. For paneer marination, take a bowl and add 30 grams of paneer cubes, curd, chaat masala, garlic paste, lemon juice, red chilli powder, and coriander powder. Mix it well.

3. Take another pan and add marinated paneer to it without any oil. Add chopped coriander leaves and sauté until the paneer is dried out.

4. Transfer this paneer to another pan where our vegetables are being sautéed and mix well.

5. Next, take 1 wheat roti and apply 1 tsp of green chutney to it.

6. Now, fill the roti with as much filling as possible and roll it. Cut it in half and enjoy!

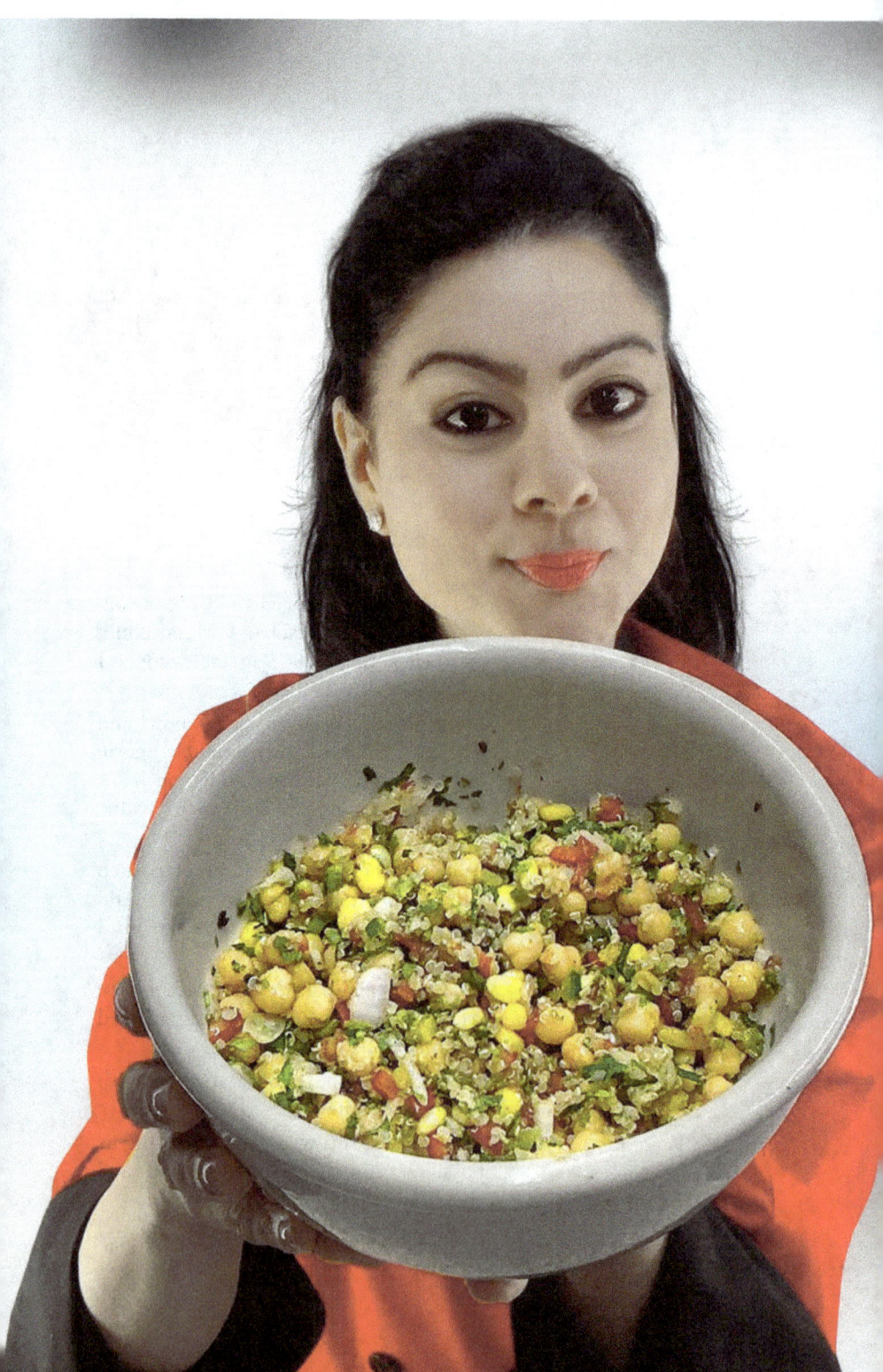

QUINOA CHICKPEA SALAD

Who says salads are boring? There's always a way to make everything interesting. Like this 180 calories per 100 grams recipe has made this quinoa chickpea salad interesting. Relish this in your weight loss journey. It's loaded with protein, fibre and carbohydrates.

INGREDIENTS:

- 50 grams boiled and strained quinoa
- 50 grams soaked and boiled white chickpeas
- 1.5 tbsp boiled sweet corn
- 1.5 tbsp finely chopped tomato
- 1.5 tbsp finely chopped onion
- Approximately 1-1.5 tbsp finely chopped green capsicum
- Approximately 1-1.5 tbsp yellow bell pepper
- Approximately 1-1.5 tbsp red bell pepper
- Approximately 1-1.5 tbsp chopped coriander leaves
- 1/2 tsp flaxseeds
- 1 tsp olive oil
- 1 tbsp white vinegar
- 1 tsp black pepper
- Salt according to your taste
- 1 tsp mustard sauce
- Half a lemon

DIRECTIONS:

1. In a bowl, add 50 grams of boiled quinoa, white chickpeas and sweet corn.
2. Next, add finely chopped tomato, onion, capsicum, red bell pepper, yellow bell pepper,
3. coriander leaves and flaxseeds.
4. For the dressing, take a bowl and add olive oil, white vinegar, black pepper powder, salt, and mustard sauce. Then squeeze half a lemon into it and mix well.
5. Spread the dressing all over the salad, mix it well and enjoy!

Note:

- Only add dressing to the salad right before consuming it. Don't add it before.

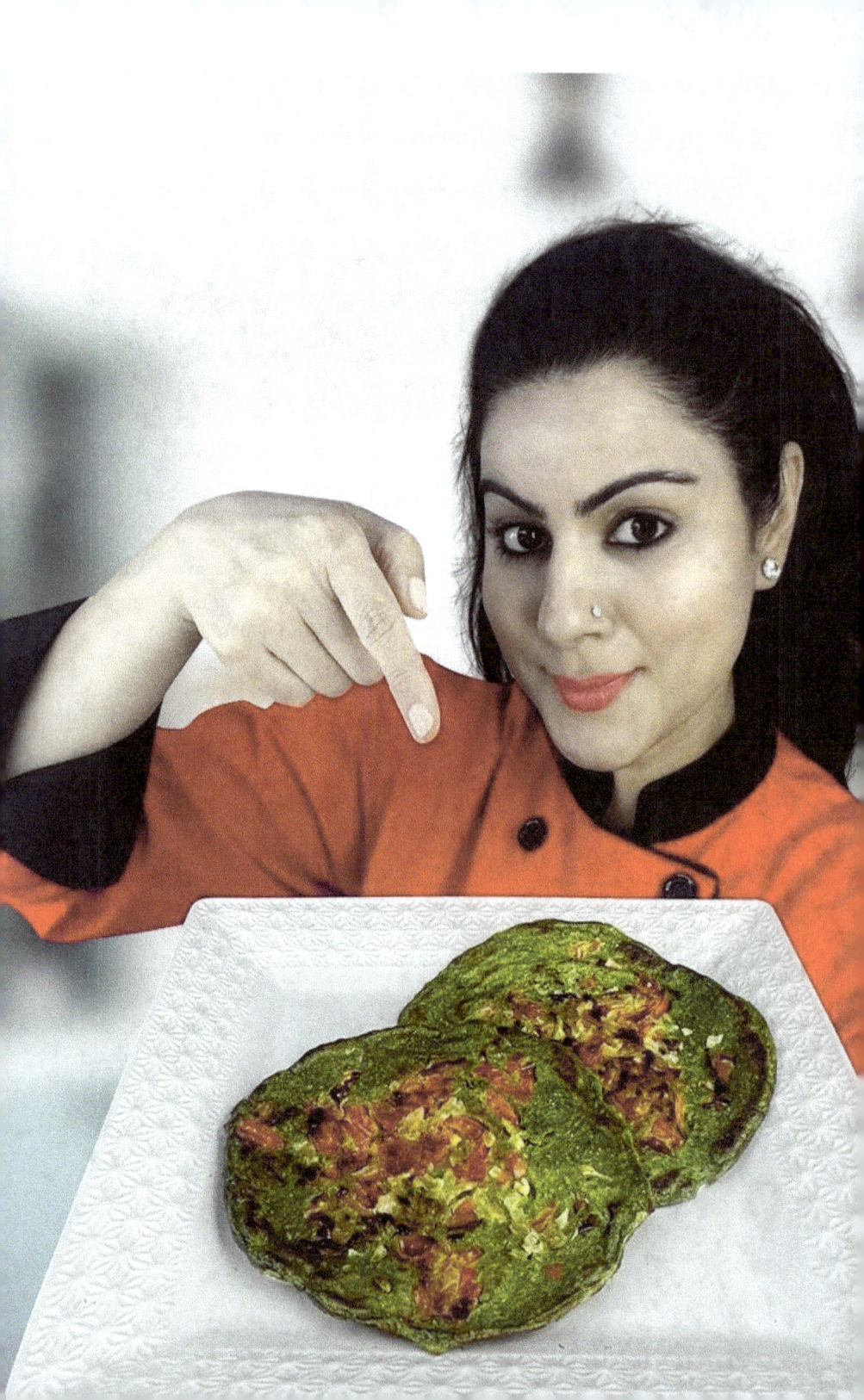

SPINACH & SPROUTS UTTAPAM

Craving for south Indian food? Then this recipe is perfect for you! Try our exceptional spinach and sprouts uttapam recipe. It's only 40 calories per uttapam. It's perfect to satisfy your craving and the taste is just incredible. Sure, try this!

INGREDIENTS:

- 100 grams spinach
- 100 grams sprouts
- 3 tbsp oats powder
- 1/2 tsp fennel seeds
- 1/2 tsp carom seeds
- A pinch of asafoetida (hing)
- 1 green chilli
- 1 tsp coriander powder
- 1/2 in ginger
- Salt according to your taste
- 1 tsp finely chopped onion
- 1 tsp finely chopped tomato

DIRECTIONS:

1. In a blender, add spinach, sprouts, oats powder, fennel seeds, carom seeds, a pinch of asafoetida, coriander powder, green chilli, ginger, salt and a little water. Blend until smooth.

2. Next, pour half of the batter into the non-stick pan and spread it a little with the help of a spoon.

3. Add some finely chopped onion and tomato to it. Cook until the spinach and sprouts Uttapam is crispy from both sides.

4. Transfer it to a plate. Eat hot and enjoy!

STUFFED ALOO PARANTHA

Who doesn't love aloo parantha? It's the perfect answer to all our needs. You just can't resist it! Try this recipe and it will bring all your childhood memories back! It's only 187 calories per parantha. You can relish it comfortably in your weight loss journey.

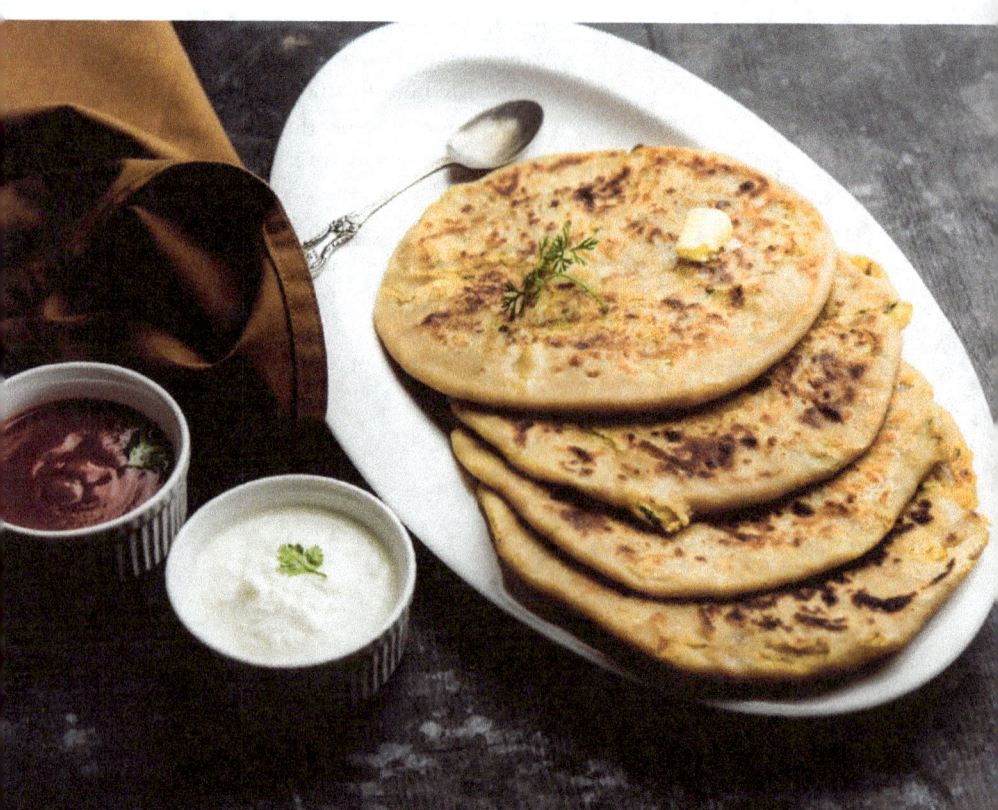

INGREDIENTS:

For filling:
- 1/2 boiled potato
- 1 tbsp boiled peas
- 1 tbsp chopped fenugreek leaves (methi leaves)
- 1 tsp chopped coriander leaves
- 1/2 tsp green chilli (roundels)
- Salt according to your taste
- 1/4 tsp garam masala
- 1/2 tsp raw mango powder (amchur)
- 1/2 tsp red chilli powder
- 1/4 tsp roasted carom seeds
- 1/4 tsp roasted cumin seeds
- 1/4 tsp roasted coriander seeds
- 1/2 tsp grated ginger
- 1 tsp ghee

For parantha:
- Whole wheat
- Water

DIRECTIONS:

1. Take a bowl and add boiled potato, boiled peas, fenugreek leaves, coriander leaves, and green chillies.
2. Next, add salt, garam masala, raw mango powder, red chilli powder, roasted carom seeds, roasted cumin seeds, roasted coriander seeds, and grated ginger.
3. Mix all the ingredients well.
4. Make a normal roti dough and roll 2 thin rotis.
5. Put the stuffing inside rolled roti and cover it with another rolled roti.
6. Take a pan and apply 1 tsp of ghee. Put your stuffed aloo parantha over it.
7. Cook, until it turns crispy from both sides and your stuffed aloo parantha is ready. Enjoy!

STUFFED PARANTHA

Why go out to eat paranthas when you can make the perfect one at your place? Try this 175 calories stuffed parantha recipe from Natasha Mohan and you'll not be able to stop licking your finger. It's that delicious!

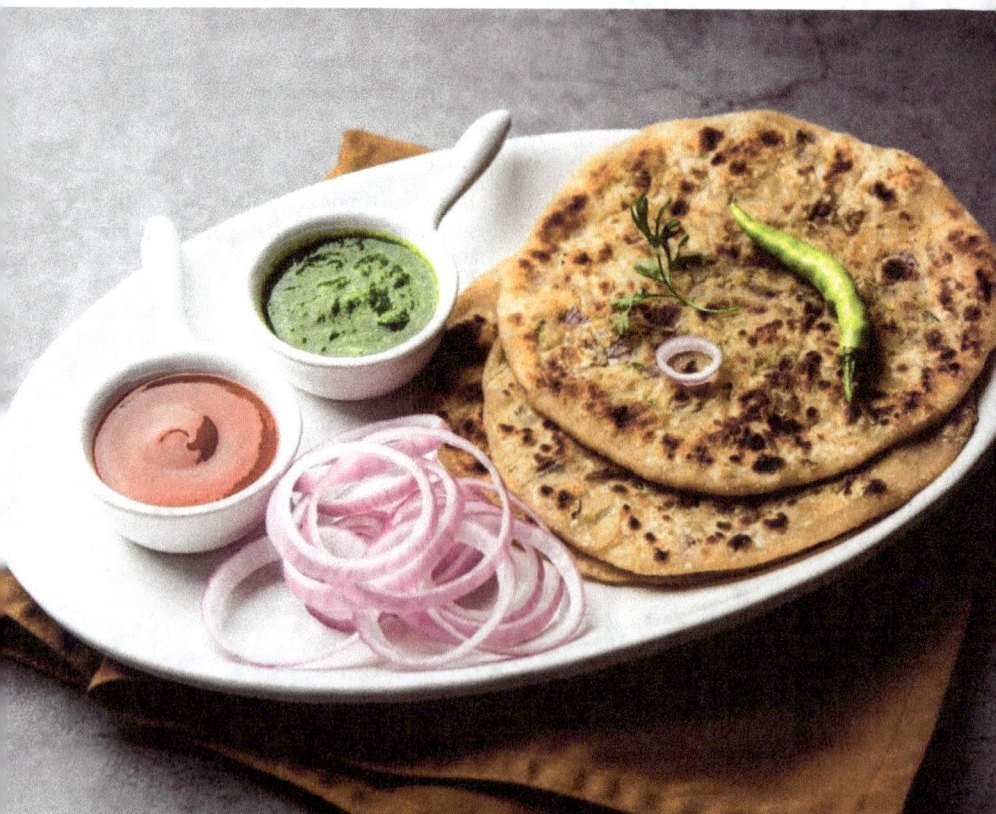

INGREDIENTS:

- 2 tbsp grated bottle gourd (lauki)
- 1 tbsp finely chopped coriander leaves
- 1 chopped green chilli (seedless) (optional)
- 1 tbsp finely chopped onion
- 1 tsp coriander powder
- 1/2 tsp roasted Carom seeds (ajwain)
- 1/2 tsp cumin seeds
- 1 tsp raw mango
- Salt according to your taste
- 1/2 cup oats powder
- 1/2 cup wheat bran flour
- 1/2 cup water
- 1/2 tsp ghee

DIRECTIONS:

1. In a bowl, add grated bottle gourd, chopped coriander leaves, green chillies and onions.
2. Next, add coriander powder, carom seeds, cumin seeds, raw mango powder and salt.
3. Now add oats powder, wheat bran flour, and water. Start mixing it with the help of a spoon.
4. It will become like a thick paste.
5. With light hands, take the dough and start spreading it and give it a parantha shape with your hands only.
6. Next, take a non-stick pan and apply some ghee on it and put the parantha over it.
7. Cook from both sides until crispy. Serve hot and enjoy!

TAWA PULAO

What's better than a plate full of scrumptious tawa pulao for your lunch? Add a lot of vegetables and you're good to go! Devour it with a bowl of curd and bliss! You can relish it comfortably because it's only 186 calories.

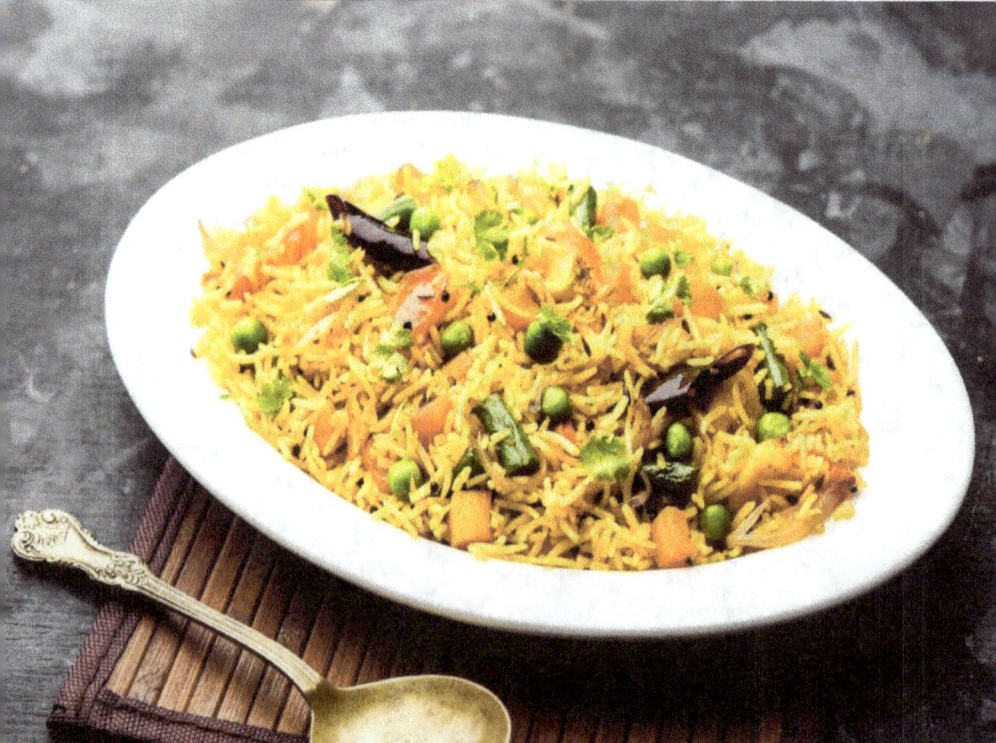

INGREDIENTS:

- 1 tsp oil
- Half cinnamon stick
- 6-7 Whole black pepper kernels
- 1/2 tsp cumin seeds
- Pinch of fenugreek seeds
- 1/2 tsp coriander seeds
- 1 tsp green chillies (chopped roundels)
- 1 tsp finely chopped garlic
- 1 tsp thinly sliced ginger julienne
- 1 tbsp finely chopped onion
- 1 tbsp finely chopped tomato
- 1 tbsp chopped beans
  1 tbsp finely chopped carrots
- 1 tbsp boiled peas
- 30-40 grams boiled chickpeas
- Salt according to your taste
- 1/2 tsp red chilli powder
- A pinch of garam masala
- 1 tsp coriander powder
- 1 tsp raw mango powder (amchur)
- 1 tsp pao bhaji masala
- 1 tbsp finely chopped coriander leaves
- 1 cup boiled rice

DIRECTIONS:

1. Take a pan and add 1 tsp of oil. Heat the oil for 2- 3 minutes.

2. Next, add cinnamon stick, black pepper kernels, cumin seeds, a pinch of fenugreek seeds, coriander seeds, and green chillies. Let the spices cook for about 2-3 minutes on low flame until they crackle.

3. Then add chopped garlic and ginger slices.

4. Now add chopped onions and sauté them until they are golden brown.

5. Then add chopped tomatoes and sauté for 2-3 minutes until the tomatoes are soft.

6. Next, add chopped beans, carrots, boiled peas and boiled chickpeas. Cook until all the vegetables are roasted. Don't overcook the vegetables. Keep them crunchy.

7. Now, add salt, red chilli powder, a pinch of garam masala and coriander powder. To make it tangy, add raw mango powder and pao bhaji masala.

8. Now add coriander leaves and boiled rice. Mix properly.

9. Transfer the pulao to the plate. Serve hot and Enjoy!

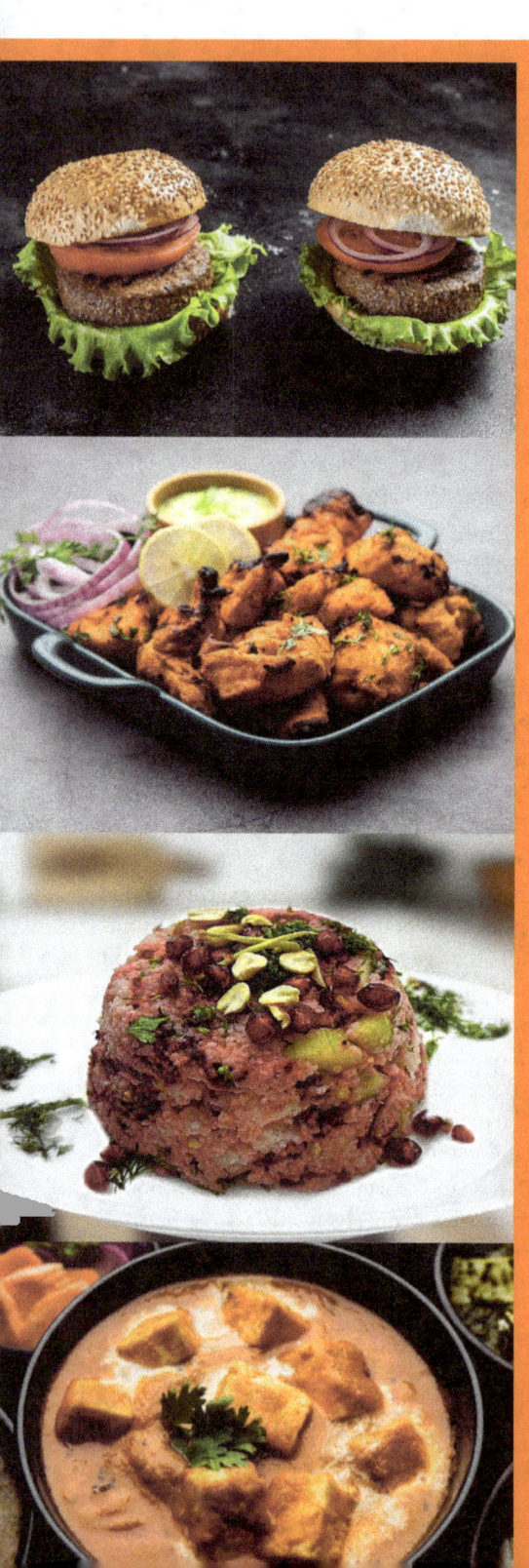

DINNER

Have you ever heard of the phrase devour breakfast like a ruler, lunch like a prince and dinner like an indigent? Well, many people think that dinner is not a vital meal of the day, and that's where they are wrong. We all know that breakfast is significant for our health, but a healthy and light dinner is also the perfect and crucial way to end the day. It enhances the functioning of our body. A healthy and nourishing dinner can help in boosting the metabolism aiding in our weight loss process.

Often with our busy schedules, we skip our dinner or consume it very late. But it's entirely against our health. Losing weight or gaining weight is related to the timing of the dinner you consume. So, try to devour your dinner between 6-8 PM, and don't stretch it after that. Because the late you eat your dinner, the more it will affect your health.

But now comes the question of what to eat for dinner that helps in losing weight. Food that is delicious and filling. Well, we have got you all covered! We have come up with surprising and exciting slim-waist dinner recipes that are so nourishing yet delicious that you'll love them. We have food for all your needs. Be it a burger craving, or you want something light and refreshing like a salad. We have all.

These recipes are so unique and different from the basic dal chawal, and you'll be amazed at how these recipes taste. You won't even realise that they are healthy recipes, and you'll be able to lose weight effortlessly with these recipes. So now you wouldn't have to think about what to cook for dinner that aids in weight loss. You can comfortably relish your dinner with these recipes as they aren't only delicious but are quick to make too!

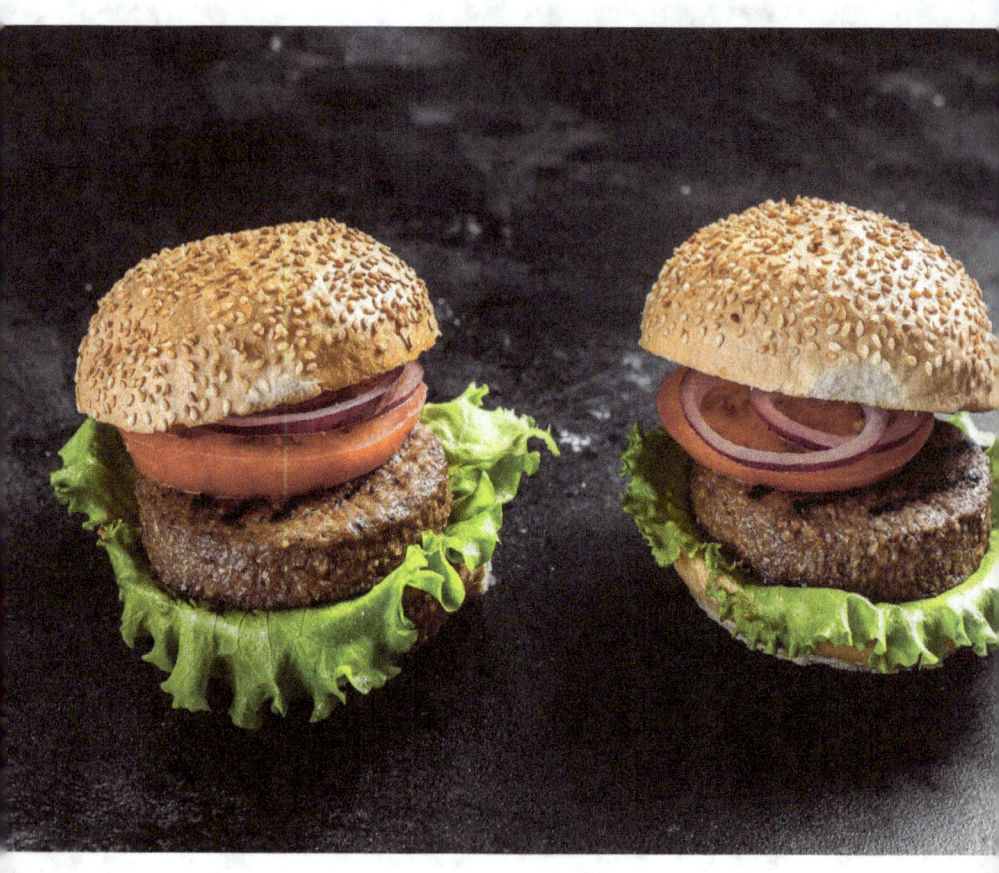

BURGER

Why go to McDonald's, when you can make one at your home? Try this amazing only 250 calories burger recipe from Natasha Mohan and satisfy your burger craving.

INGREDIENTS:

- 1 tsp oil
- 1/2 tsp cumin seeds
- 1 tbsp finely chopped onion
- 1 tbsp finely chopped beans
- 1 tbsp finely chopped carrot
- 1 cup soya chunks (soaked in lukewarm water for 30 minutes)
- 1/2 tsp red chilli powder
- 1 tsp coriander powder
- 1 tsp raw mango powder (amchur)
- 1/4 tsp garam masala
- 1 onion rings
- 1 whole wheat burger buns
- 1 tsp mustard sauce
- 1/2 tomato roundels slices
- Olives (optional)
- Jalapeños (optional)

DIRECTIONS:

1. In a frying pan, add oil, cumin seeds, finely chopped onion, beans, and carrots. Sauté the vegetables for 1-2 minutes.

2. Now take soaked soya chunks, squeeze all their water and add to the pan.

3. Next, add red chilli powder, coriander powder, raw mango powder, and garam masala. Mix all the ingredients well. Let it cook for a few minutes.

4. Transfer the soya and vegetable mixture into a bowl and keep it aside for cooling. After it's cooled, transfer the mixture into a blender and grind it until it comes to a coarse texture.

5. Give the mixture a patty shape and put it in a non-stick pan. Let it cook until turn brown and crispy on both sides.

6. Now, take 1 onion and cut it into roundels. (Onion rings) In a frying pan, sauté the onion roundels for a few minutes. Keep on stirring them.

7. Next, in a frying pan, lightly toast the wheat buns and apply 1 tsp mustard sauce over the plain side of the bun.

8. Add lots of lettuce leaves, tomato roundels, soya tikki, sautéed onion rings, olives, and jalapeños. Cover it with another wheat bun and enjoy!

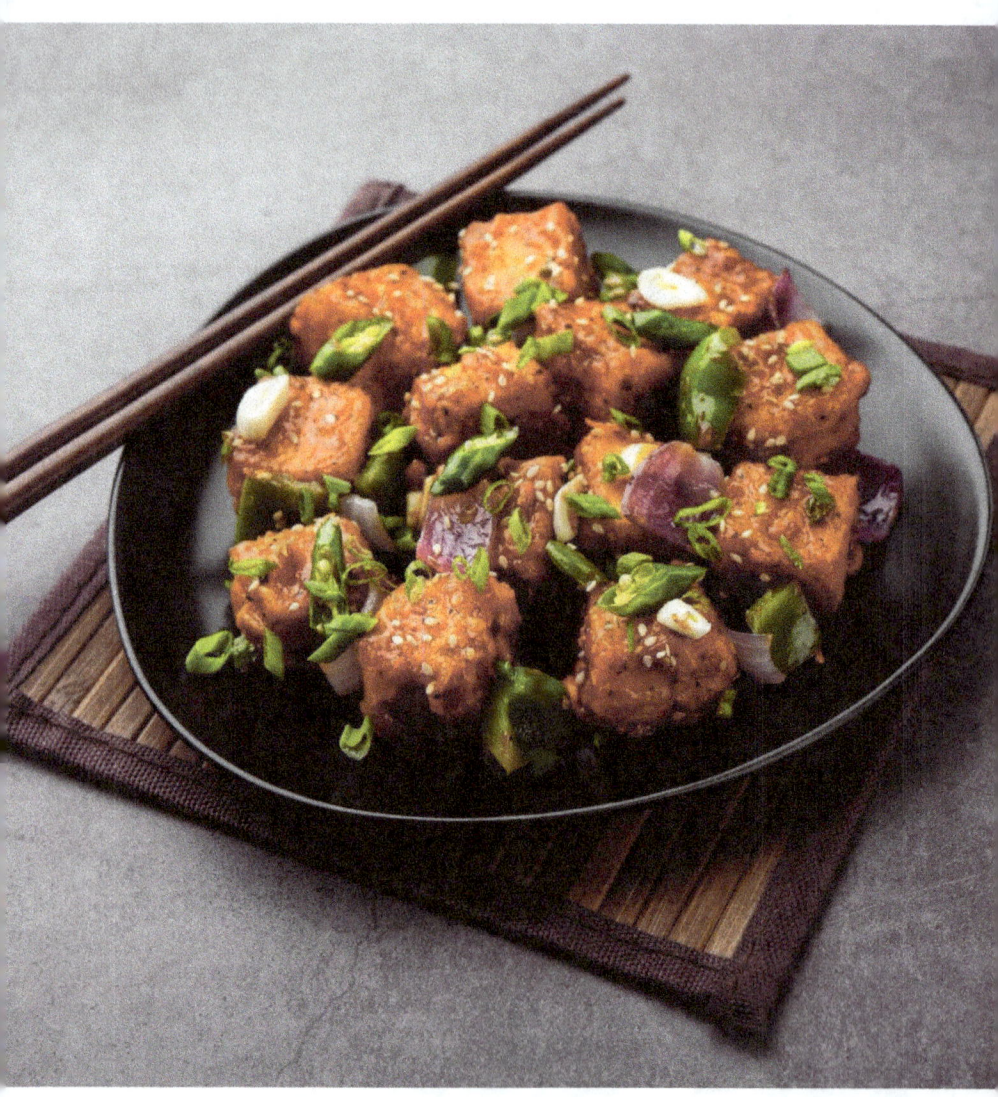

CHILLY PANEER

Chilly paneer can never go wrong! Especially when made with such a healthy recipe. Low in calories, high in protein! Pair it with some boiled rice or roti and enjoy! It only has 150-180 calories!

INGREDIENTS:

- 1 tsp oil
- 1 tbsp chopped garlic
- 1-inch ginger stick paste
- 100 grams paneer (chopped into cubes)
- 2-3 pieces slit green chillies (seedless)
- 1 small onion diced
- 1/2 yellow bell pepper diced
- 1/2 green capsicum diced
- 1 tbsp soy sauce
- 1 tbsp red chilli sauce
- 1.5 tbsp ketchup
- 1 tbsp vinegar
- Salt according to your taste
- 1/2 tsp white pepper powder

GARNISH:

- Sesame seeds

DIRECTIONS:

1. In a frying pan add 1 tsp oil, chopped garlic and ginger paste. Sauté until the rawness of ginger and garlic vanishes for 1-2 minutes on low flame.
2. Next, add paneer cubes and cook until the paneer gets all crispy.
3. Now, add slit green chillies, and toss them for about 2-3 minutes.
4. Next, add diced onion, yellow bell pepper, and green capsicum.
5. Now, add soy sauce, red chilli sauce, ketchup, and 1 tbsp vinegar.
6. Add salt and white pepper powder and transfer it to a bowl, Sprinkle with sesame seeds over and enjoy!

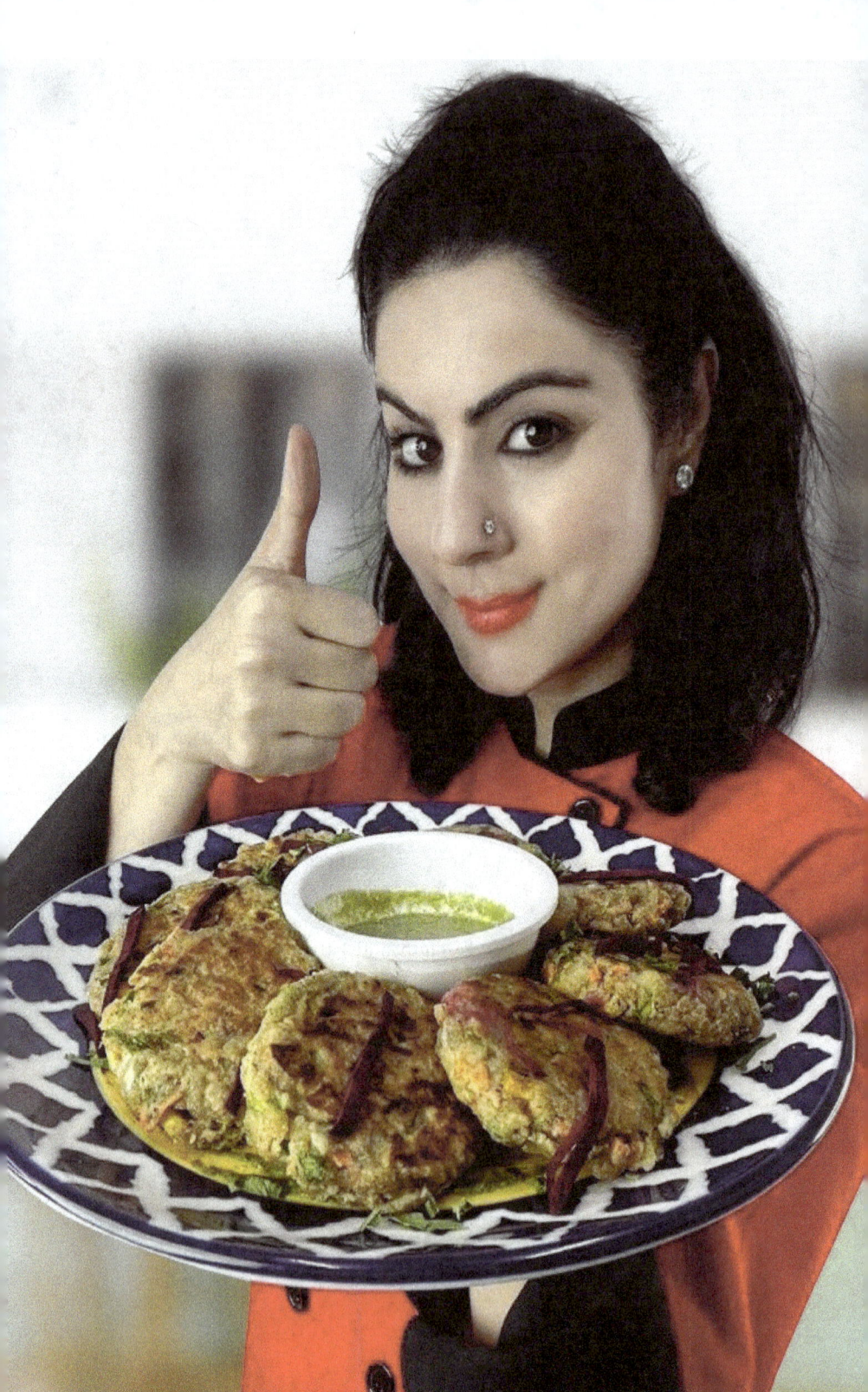

DAHI KE KEBAB

Are you looking for a recipe that helps you make quick and easy dahi ke kebabs? Here's one with only 35 calories per piece! Low in calories and so easy to make!

INGREDIENTS:

- 100 grams hung curd*
- 2-3 tbsp finely chopped onion
- 2-3 tbsp finely chopped carrot
- 1-3 tbsp finely chopped capsicum
- 2-3 tbsp finely chopped cabbage
- 6-7 finely chopped coriander leaves
- Salt according to your taste
- 1 tsp red chilli powder
- 1/4 tsp garam masala
- 1/4 tsp cumin powder
- 1-2 tsp coriander powder
- 1/2 tsp black pepper powder
- Ragi flour* 1 tbsp oil

GARNISH:

- Beetroot juliennes

Note:

*Take a muslin cloth and strain your normal curd from it.

*If you don't have ragi flour, you can take any other millet flour.

DIRECTIONS:

1. Take a bowl and add 100 grams of hung curd, chopped onions, carrots, cabbage and capsicum to it.
2. Now add finely chopped coriander leaves, salt, red chilli powder, garam masala, cumin powder, coriander powder, and black pepper powder to it.
3. Mix it well so that everything mixes well.
4. Now keep the mixture in the refrigerator for 5- 10 minutes.
5. After 5-10 minutes, give this mixture a nice tikki shape.
6. After giving a tikki shape, refrigerate or freeze it for 5-10 minutes.
7. Take some ragi flour into a plate and coat the kebabs with it properly. After coating the kebabs, refrigerate these for 5-10 minutes.
8. Take a pan and spread the oil on it. We'll shallow fry the kebabs. Put the kebabs in the pan and cook until they are golden brown and crispy on both sides.
9. Turn these gently because they are very soft.
10. Transfer these kebabs to a plate and garnish with beetroot juliennes. And, voilà, dahi kebabs are ready! Enjoy!

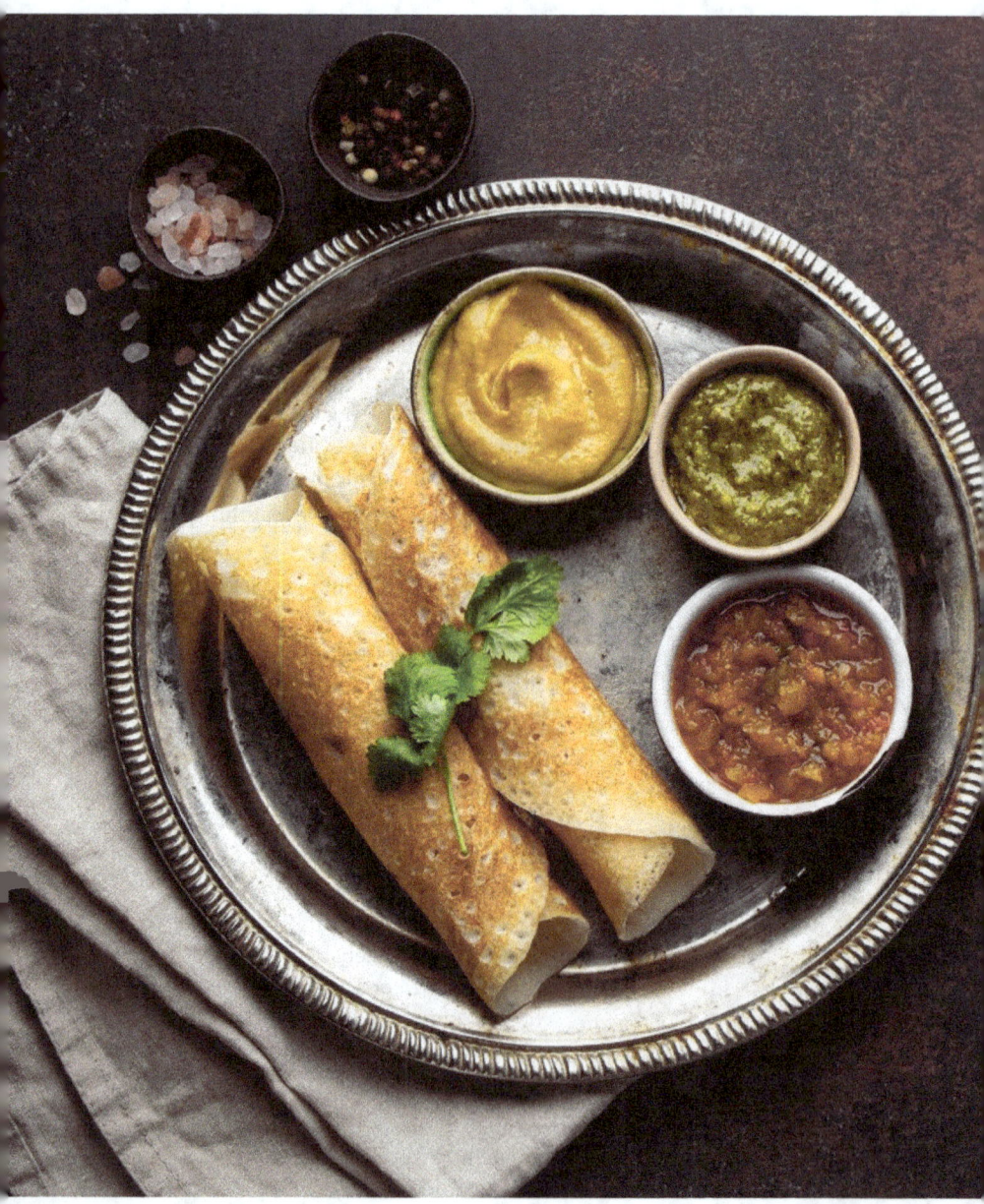

OATS & DAL DOSA

What's better than cooking a dosa at your place that is completely healthy, and you can devour it in your weight loss journey without being stressed about gaining weight? Try this delectable, oats and dal dosa recipe from Natasha Mohan and we assure you, you'll love it! It's only 165 calories per dosa!

INGREDIENTS:

- 30 grams yellow moong dal
- 30 grams oats
- Water 1/2 glass
- Salt according to your taste
- 1.5 tbsp thinly sliced onion
- 1.5 tbsp thinly sliced cabbage
- 1.5 tbsp thinly sliced capsicum
- 1.5 tbsp thinly sliced beans
- 1.5 tbsp thinly sliced carrot
- 30 grams paneer (diced into thin slices)
- 1 tsp chopped coriander leaves
- 1 tsp black pepper powder
- 1 tsp coriander powder
- 1 tsp raw mango powder (amchur)
- 1/2 tsp oil (for cooking)

DIRECTIONS:

1. In a bowl add 30 grams of moong dal and wash it until the water is clear.
2. Next, add 30 grams of oats and 1/2 glass of water. Let the dal and oats soak for about 30 minutes to 1 hour.
3. If you own a microwave, you can also microwave this mixture for 1-2 minutes to get it puffy.
4. Transfer this mixture into a blender, add a pinch of salt and blend until a thick paste is formed.
5. Transfer the paste into a bowl.
6. For dosa filling, in a non-stick pan without adding oil, add thinly sliced onion, cabbage, capsicum, capsicum, beans, paneer slices, and chopped coriander leaves.
7. Now, add black pepper powder, coriander powder, and raw mango powder. Dry roast the vegetables until the paneer is crispy and the vegetables are cooked.
8. Brush a little oil into the frying pan and spread the dosa batter over it. Don't flip the dosa, let it cook for 3-4 and get it crispy.
9. Put the filling inside the dosa and fold it.
10. Serve hot and enjoy!

PANEER MAKHANI

Love paneer makhani but not being able to relish it due to the weight hassles? You'll love this 148 calories recipe! Our healthy twist on paneer makhani. It's so amazing that you can easily incorporate this into your weight loss journey without any stress!

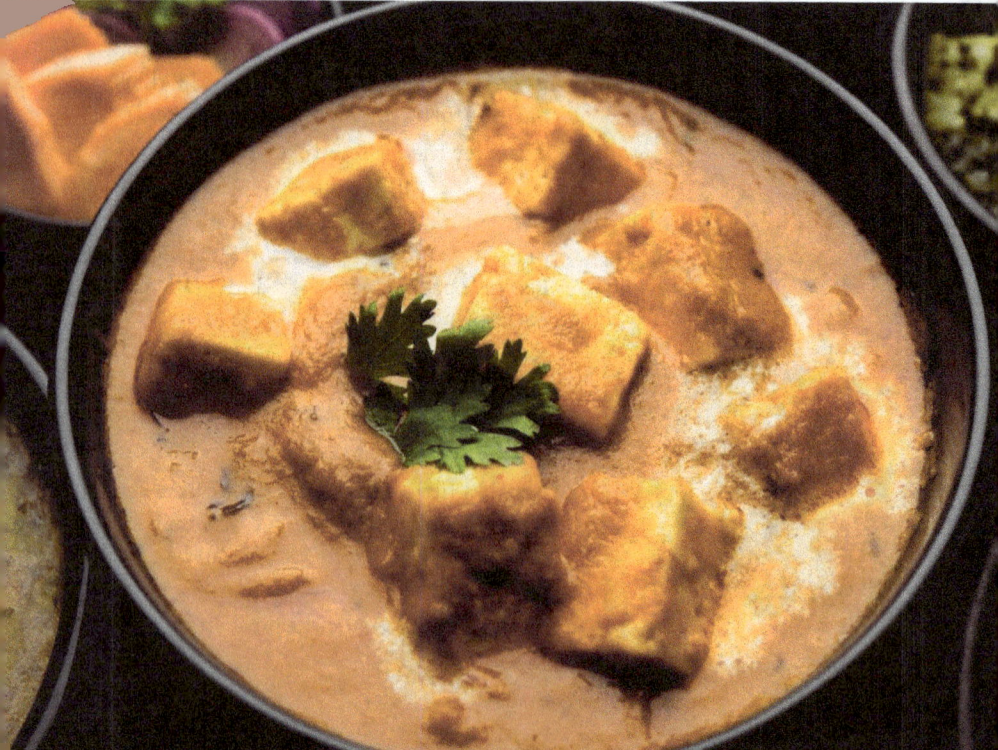

INGREDIENTS:

- 1 tsp mustard oil.
- 3-4 green chillies (slit from between)
- 1 tsp garlic paste
- 2 whole tomatoes (puréed)
- 1/2 tsp coriander powder
- Approximately 1/2-1 tsp Kashmir red chilli (for colour)
- Salt according to your taste
- 1/2 tsp kasoori methi
- Pinch of garam masala Water
- 1/2-1 tsp sugar
- 1/2 cup milk
- Approximately 5-6 paneer cubes

DIRECTIONS:

1. Take a frying pan and add 1 tsp mustard oil to it.
2. Heat it for 2-3 minutes and add green chillies and garlic paste. Cook it for 2 minutes.
3. Add tomato puree to the pan and cook it for 5- 6 minutes on low flame.
4. Then add coriander powder, Kashmiri red chilli, salt, kasoori methi and garam masala.
5. Add some water to prevent the mixture (masala) from burning. Mix it well and cook for 2 minutes.
6. Add some sugar to balance out the sourness of tomatoes and milk.
7. Then add paneer cubes to the sauce and mix it properly. Let it cook for 1 minute on low flame and enjoy!

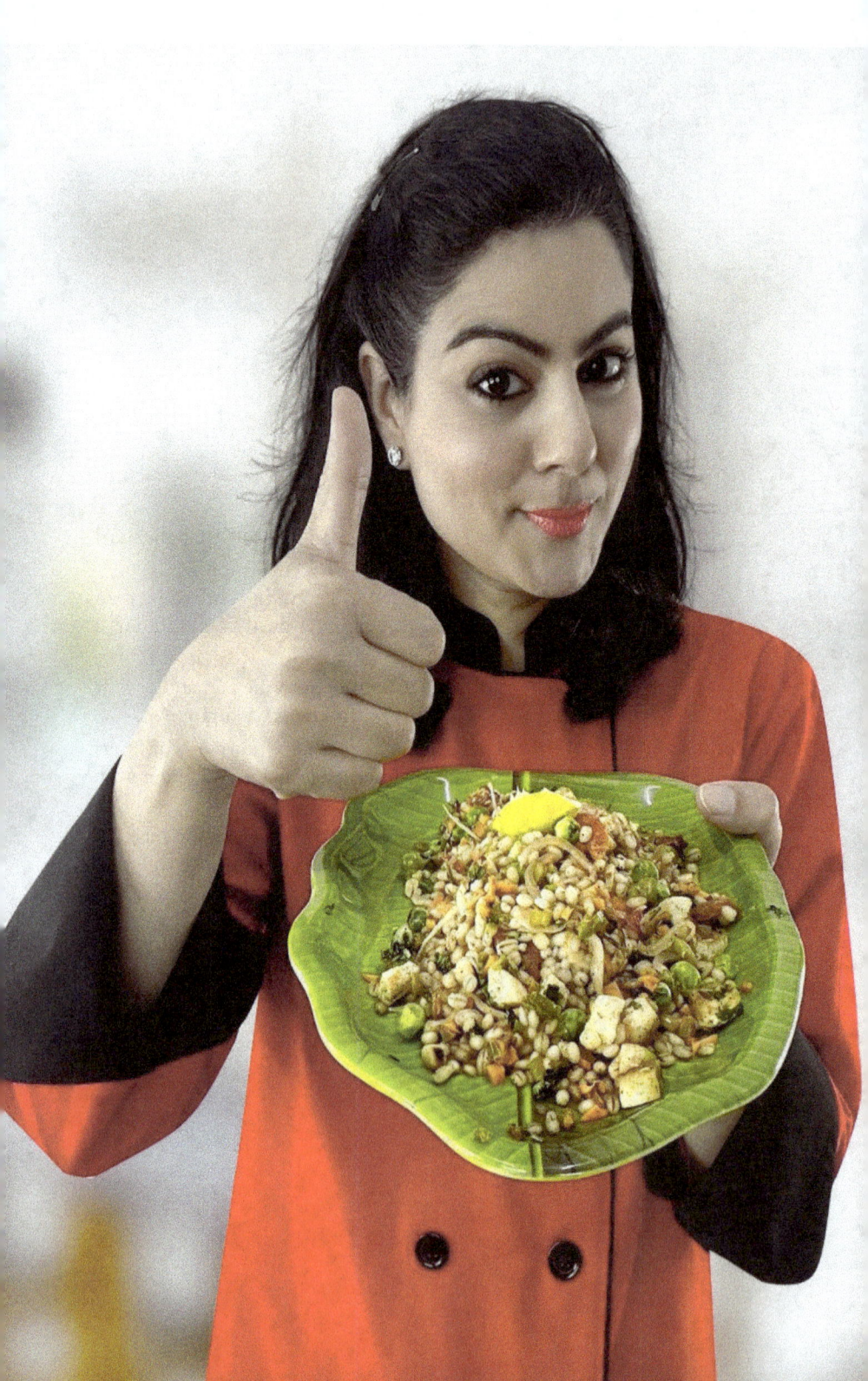

PEARL MILLET SALAD

In search of a salad? Well, try this one! Pearl millet salad with goodness of cottage cheese and veggies. It's so refreshing, so mouth-watering that you won't be able to resist! And it's only 212 calories! Amazing, right?

INGREDIENTS:

- 1/2 tsp oil
- 1 tsp cumin seeds
- 1/2 tsp coriander seeds
- 1 tsp green chilli roundels
- 1 tbsp thinly sliced onions
- 1 tbsp thinly sliced tomato
- 20 grams cottage cheese cubes (paneer)
- 20 grams boiled peas
- 20 grams finely chopped carrot
- 20 grams finely chopped capsicum
- 1/2 tsp coriander powder
- 1/2 tsp garam masala
- 1/2 tsp raw mango powder
- 1/2 tsp red chilli powder
- Salt according to your taste
- 70 grams cooked pearl millet (bajra)
- 1 tsp chopped coriander leaves
- 1 tsp peanuts

DIRECTIONS:

1. In a pan add oil, cumin seeds, coriander seeds, and green chillies. Cook until the seeds crackle.
2. Next, add onions and tomatoes. Sauté for 2-3 minutes.
3. Then add cottage cheese cubes, boiled peas, carrots, and capsicum.
4. Next, add coriander powder, garam masala, raw mango powder, red chilli powder, and salt.
5. Now add cooked pearl millet to it and cook for 2 minutes.
6. Add coriander leaves and peanuts. Mix all the ingredients well.
7. Transfer the salad to a plate and enjoy!

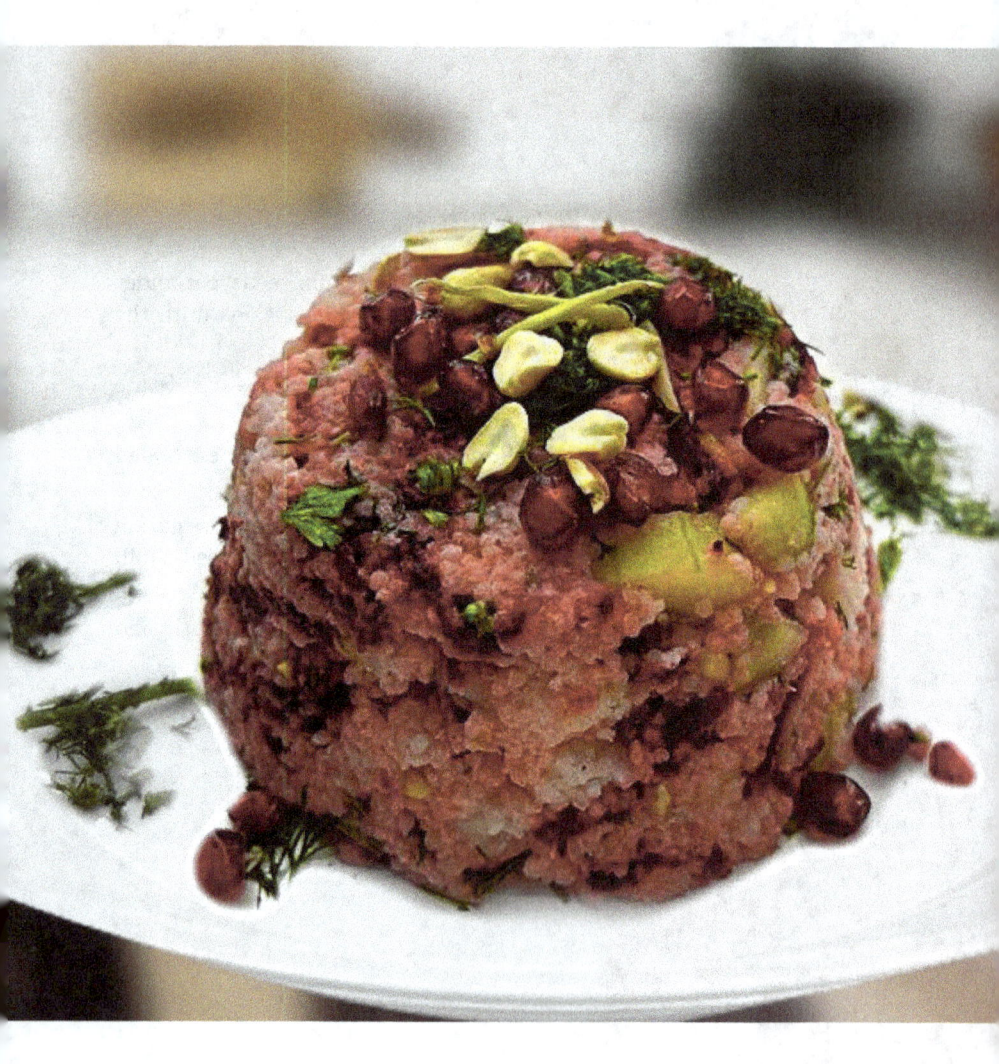

SAMA RICE SALAD

Want to have something light for dinner? This is the perfect option! Less than 100 calories of sama rice salad! Quick and easy to make with lots of protein in it. Light and filling at the same time!

INGREDIENTS:

- 30 grams boiled sama rice
- 1/2 chopped cucumber
- 1/2 chopped tomato
- 1 tbsp grated beetroot
- 1 tbsp chopped coriander leaves
- 1/2 cup curd
- Salt according to your taste
- 1 tsp cumin powder
- 1/2 tsp black pepper
- 1/2 lemon
- 1 tbsp chopped peanuts

GARNISH:

- Chopped coriander leaves
- Pomegranate seeds

DIRECTIONS:

1. In a bowl add boiled sama rice, chopped cucumber, tomato, beetroot, and coriander leaves.
2. For the dressing, take 1/2 cup of curd and add cumin powder, salt, and black pepper powder.
3. Mix the spices with curd well and spread over the salad well.
4. Next, squeeze 1/2 lemon over the salad and mix it well.
5. Now, add peanuts to it. Mix all the ingredients well.
6. Transfer the salad to a bowl and garnish it with chopped coriander leaves and pomegranate seeds. Enjoy!

VEG BIRYANI

For all biryani lovers, this recipe is a must-try. Because it's my zero oil veg biryani recipe. It contains less than 150 calories, it's super healthy yet scrumptious, and you can easily relish this in your weight loss journey too. A perfect option for dinner!

INGREDIENTS:

- 1 onion juliennes
- 30-40 grams paneer cubes
- 7-8 cauliflower florets
- Approximately chopped 1 carrot
- 20-30 grams of beans
- Approximately 1-2 chopped tomatoes and 1 cardamom (small)
- 2-3 cloves
- 5-6 black pepper
- 1/2 cinnamon
- 1 mace (javitri)
- 1 cup curd

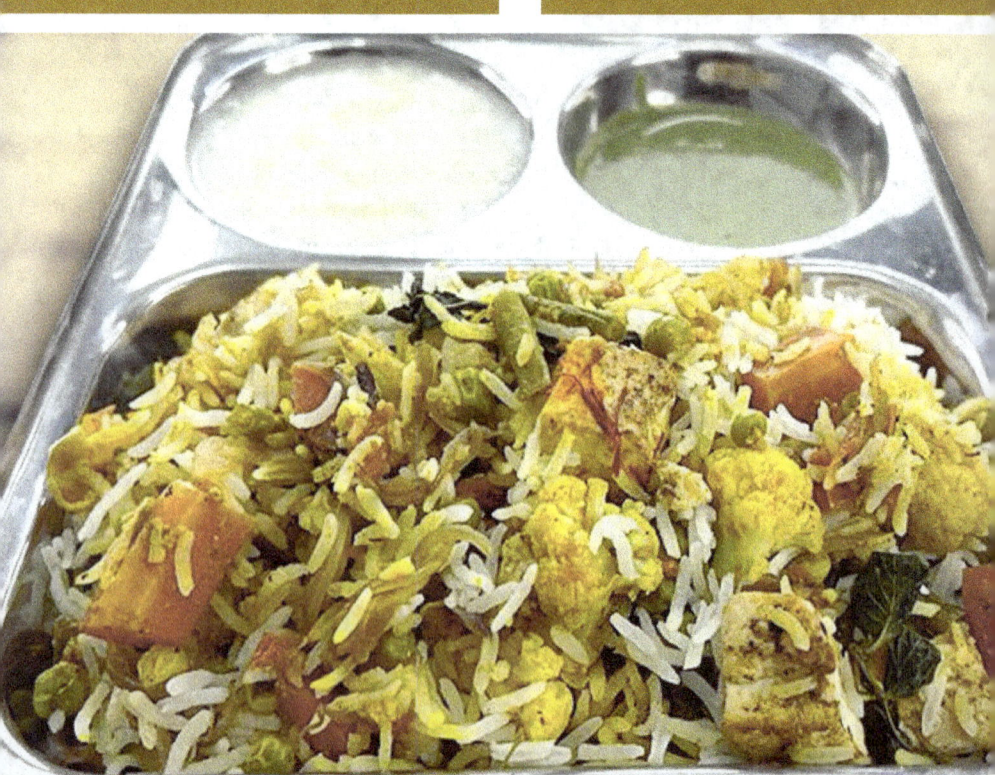

- Approximately 1-2 tsp coriander powder
- 1/2 tsp turmeric powder Salt according to your taste
- 1/4 tsp garam masala
- 1 tsp cumin powder
- 1/4 tsp red chilli powder (optional)
- 1 tsp dried fenugreek leaves powder (kasuri methi)
- 2 tbsp boiled peas
- 1 tsp ginger garlic paste
- 4-5 chopped mint leaves
- 10 tbsp boiled rice
- 2 tbsp milk Saffron

DIRECTIONS:

1. Take a non-stick pan and without adding any oil, add onions and sauté the onions for 3-4 minutes till the onions get golden brown. After sautéing the onions move them to a plate.

2. In the same pan add cottage cheese and roast them till they are brown. After roasting the cottage cheese move them to the plate.

3. Now, we'll add vegetables to the same pan. Add cauliflower florets, carrots, and beans.

4. Now, we don't have oil, that's why we'll use water to cook the vegetables. Add a little water to cook the vegetables. Cover the pan with a lid and cook it for about 2-3 minutes.

5. Now for biryani's gravy, in a pan add tomatoes, clove, cinnamon stick, black pepper, cardamom, and javitri.

6. Add a little water until the tomatoes are softened and come in gravy form. Cover it with a lid and cook for about 2-3 minutes.

7. Now, add the precooked vegetables to this mixture.

8. Now, take a bowl of curd and add coriander powder, turmeric, salt, garam masala, red chilli powder (optional) cumin powder, and dried fenugreek seeds powder.

9. Mix the spices with curd well and add them to the mixture.

10. After adding the curd, add boiled peas, and ginger garlic paste. Mix it well and let it cook till the water in the curry gets a little dried out.

11. It's time for layering now! To layer the biryani, add mint leaves and roasted onions over the vegetables.

12. Now, spread a layer of rice over the vegetables and after spreading them add roasted paneer cubes over the rice.

13. Now take 2 tbsp milk and mix some saffron in it. Spread this milk and saffron mixture over the biryani.

14. Cover it and cook it for about 5 minutes and your vegetable biryani is ready. Serve hot and Enjoy!

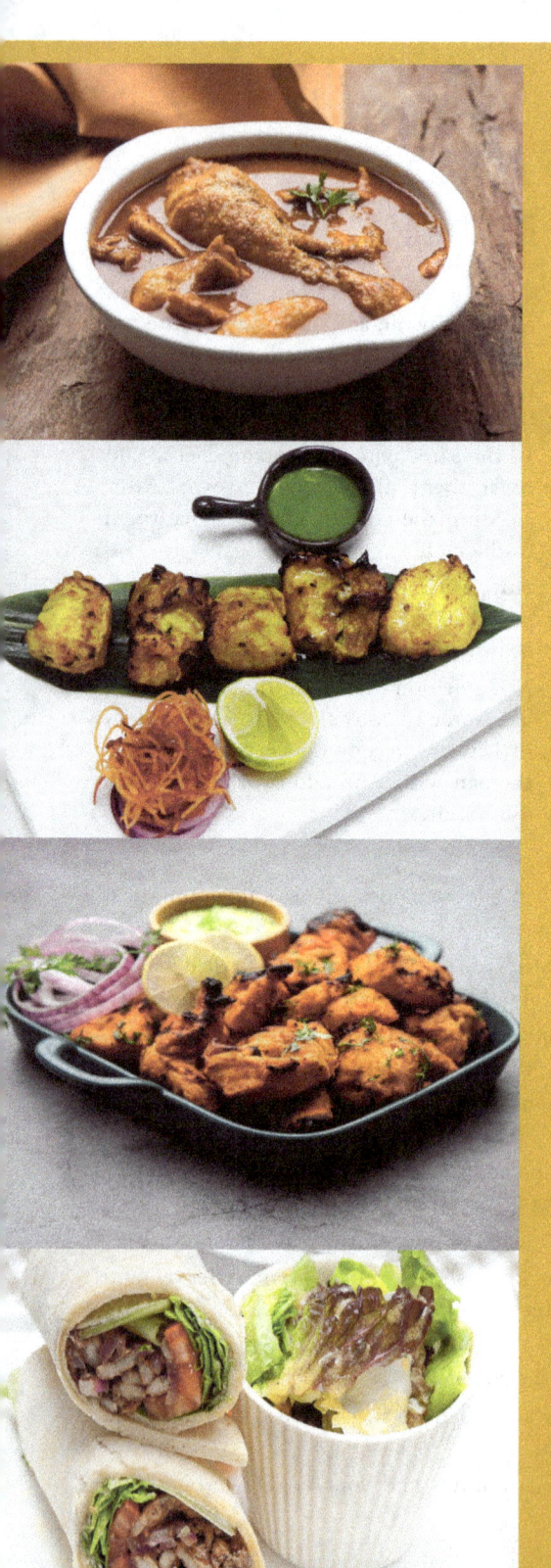

NON - VEG SPECIAL

You know protein is considered very good during your weight loss process. Many diets include more protein-based food in the weight loss journey. There's no doubt about it that protein-rich foods aid in weight loss. One of the main reasons for incorporating protein-rich food into your diet is because they are so filling that after eating them, you don't feel hungry for long. You stay full. They also help in boosting your metabolism, which also aids in weight loss. And what's better than chicken or protein to fulfil your protein requirements?

Who thought we forgot to add something special for all the meat lovers? We did not! We have added 4 Special non-vegetarian dishes that you'll love. But mostly non-vegetarian dishes require a lot of oil to cook. And consumption of a lot of oil during the weight loss journey doesn't seem like a good idea, right? So, to overcome this problem, we have got you recipes that contain only a little oil and can fulfil all your protein requirements easily. They are so flavourful and appetizing that you will not be able to resist them. Try these recipes now and fulfil all your protein requirements with our mouth-watering and healthy recipes.

CHICKEN CURRY

Want restaurant-like chicken curry at home? Here's my grandmother's recipe with my healthy twist. It's so delectable that you'll forget the restaurant's chicken curry. You get all this deliciousness in just 210 calories.

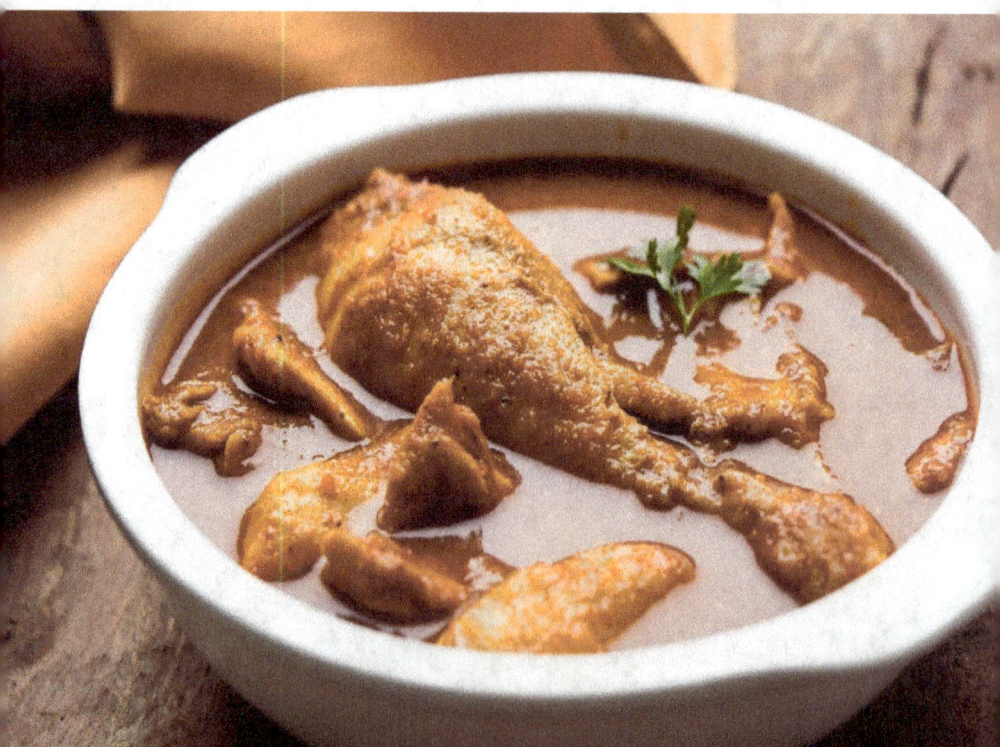

INGREDIENTS:

- 1 kg raw chicken
- 4-5 pieces of clove
- 2-3 pieces of small cardamom
- 1 piece of black cardamom
- 1 cinnamon stick
- 2-3 curry leaves
- 2-3 tsp ginger garlic paste
- 3-4 onions paste
- 3-4 tomatoes paste
- 2 tbsp coriander powder
- 1 tbsp turmeric powder
- Salt according to your taste
- 2 tbsp cumin powder
- 1 tbsp red chilli powder
- 1/4 tbsp garam masala
- Oil to cook

DIRECTIONS:

1. In a pan, add oil and cloves, cinnamon stick, small cardamom, black cardamom, curry leaves, and ginger-garlic paste. Let it cook on a low flame until the rawness of garlic vanishes.

2. Take a blender and blend 3-4 onions without water to make onion paste and transfer it into a bowl. Repeat the same process with tomato.

3. Next, add the onion paste to the pan and cover it for about 3-4 minutes on low flame.

4. Now, add salt, coriander powder, turmeric powder, red chilli powder, garam masala, and cumin powder. Mix all the ingredients well and let cook for about 3-4 minutes.

5. Cover the pan with a lid and let it cook for 7-8 minutes. Now, add tomato paste and mix it well and cover it for 7-8 minutes.

6. Transfer chicken pieces to the pan and add salt to it. Mix it well and cover it for 10-15 minutes on a low flame.

7. Transfer your chicken curry to a bowl and garnish it with chopped coriander leaves and enjoy!

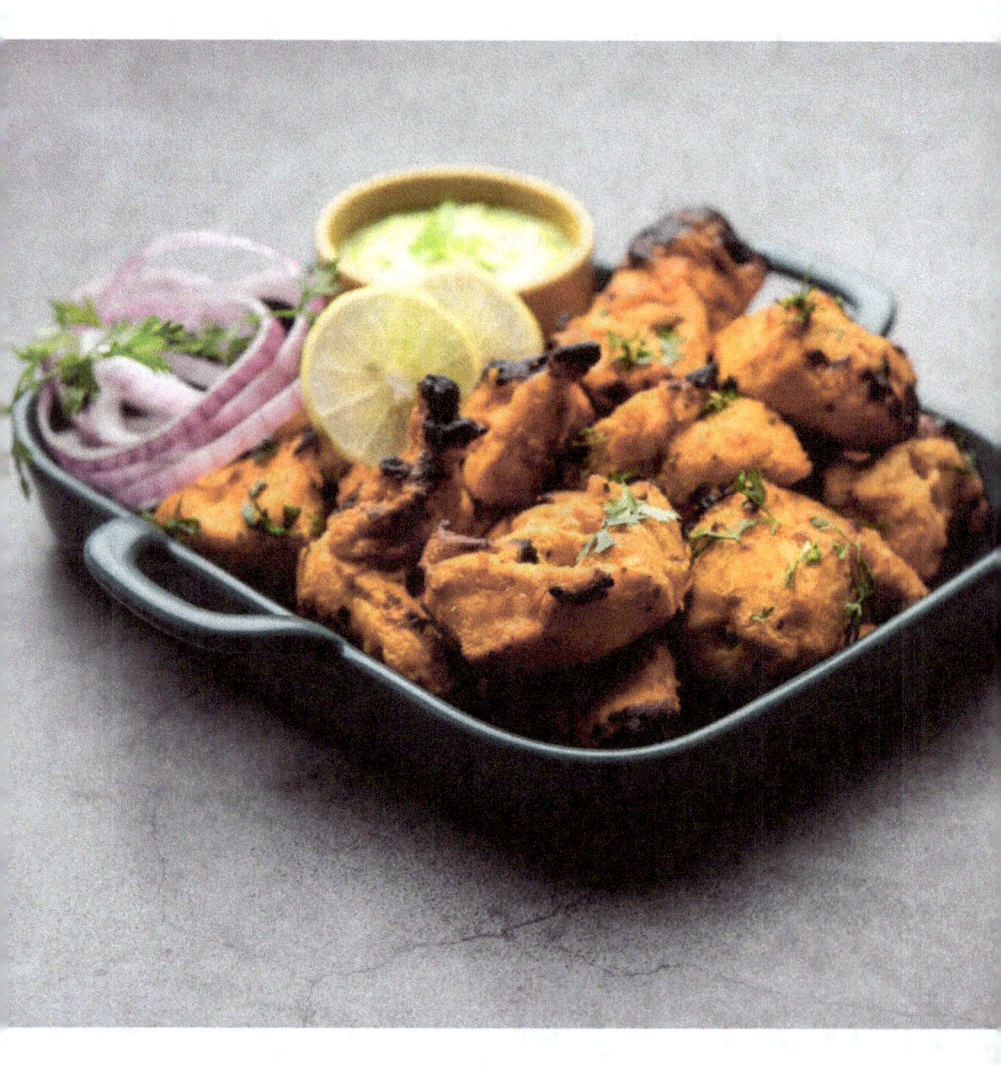

CHICKEN TIKKA

Those who are always in the mood for some appetizing chicken tikka. It's bliss on the plate and mouth! It has got all the flavours in just 121 calories!

INGREDIENTS:

- 1/2 cup curd
- 2 whole red chillies
- 5-6 minced garlic cloves
- Approximately 1/2-1 tsp fenugreek (methi daana)
- Approximately 1 tsp fennel seeds (saunf)
- 1 tsp Kashmiri red chilli powder
- Salt according to your taste
- 1 onion thin julienne slices
- 50 grams of chicken breast (chopped into pieces)
- 5-6 chopped coriander leaves

DIRECTIONS:

1. For chicken marination, take a bowl and add 1/2 cup curd to it. Whisk it properly.

2. Add whole red chillies, chopped garlic, fenugreek, fennel seeds, Kashmiri red chilli powder, salt and sliced onions. Mix it well.

3. Now, add chicken pieces to the marination. Coat the chicken with marination properly and keep it in the refrigerator for about 1-2 hours.

4. Take a non-stick pan and add your mixture to it without adding any oil.

5. Cook it on a low flame for 10-20 minutes.

6. Move your chicken tikka to the plate and sprinkle some freshly chopped coriander leaves over it and enjoy!

MEXICAN CHICKEN WRAP

In the mood for some chicken wrap? Try this amazing, only 160 calories Mexican chicken wrap recipe. It has got all the flavours you need. It's so appetizing that you'll want it again and again.

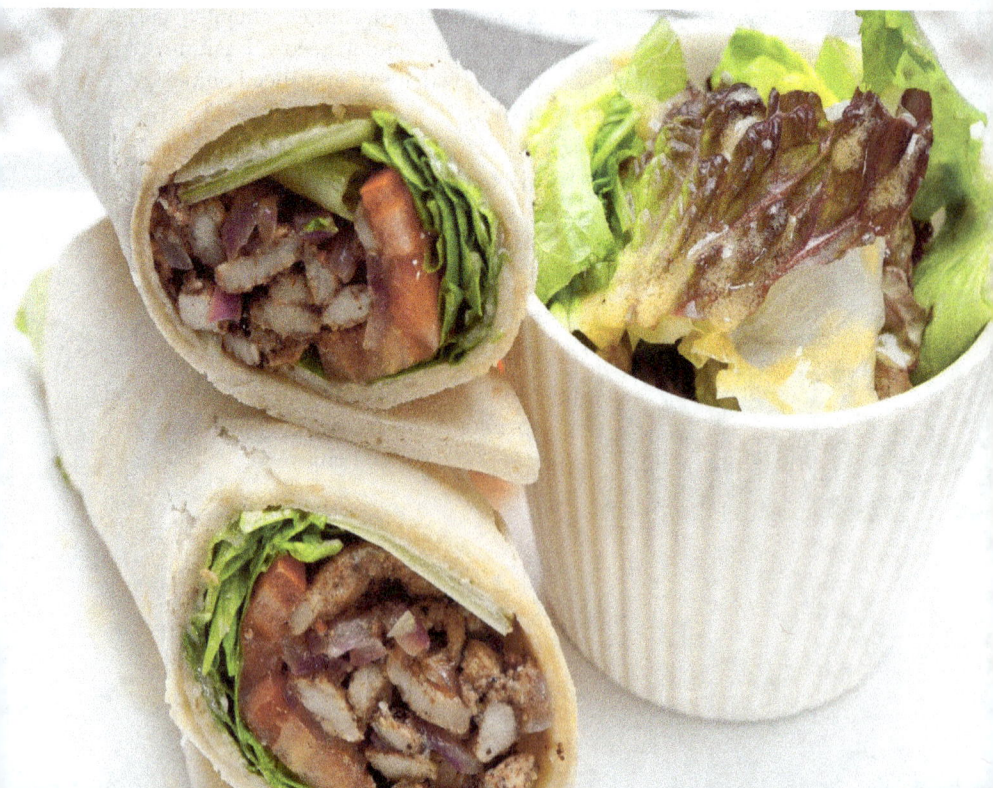

INGREDIENTS:

- 1 tsp oil
- 1/2 tsp garlic paste
- 1/2 tsp cumin seeds
- 1 tbsp finely chopped onion
- 1 tbsp finely chopped carrot
- 1 tbsp finely chopped beans
- 1 tbsp finely chopped mushrooms
- 100 grams of minced chicken
- 1 tbsp finely chopped capsicum
- 1 tbsp finely chopped yellow bell pepper
- 1 tbsp finely chopped red bell pepper
- 2 tomatoes puree
- 1/2 tsp black pepper powder
- 1 tsp cinnamon powder
- 1/4 tsp garam masala
- Salt according to your taste
- 1 tsp coriander powder
- 1/2 tsp Kashmiri red chilli powder
- 1 wheat tortilla
- 1 tsp salsa sauce
- 1 tsp sour cream
- Lettuce

DIRECTIONS:

1. In a non-stick frying pan, add 1 tsp of oil, garlic paste, and cumin seeds. Sauté until cumin seeds start to crackle.

2. Next, add finely chopped onion, carrot, beans, and mushrooms. Sauté the vegetables on high flame for about 30-40 seconds. Next, cover it and let it cook on low flame for about 1-2 minutes.

3. Now, add minced chicken, finely chopped capsicum, yellow bell pepper, red bell pepper, and tomato puree. Mix all the ingredients well. Cover it and let it cook on low flame for 5-6 minutes.

4. Next, add black pepper powder, cinnamon powder, garam masala, salt, coriander powder, and Kashmiri red chilli powder. Mix all the ingredients well. Cover it and let it cook.

5. Take 1 wheat tortilla and a spoonful of our chicken mixture, 1 tsp salsa sauce, sour cream, and lettuce.

6. Now, fold the tortilla tightly like a roll. Cut it from between and enjoy!

TANDOORI FISH

For the fish lovers! We have got a special recipe for you all as well! Try this impeccable fish tikka recipe. Only 270 calories! High in protein and filled with flavours! So easy to make that you'll love it!

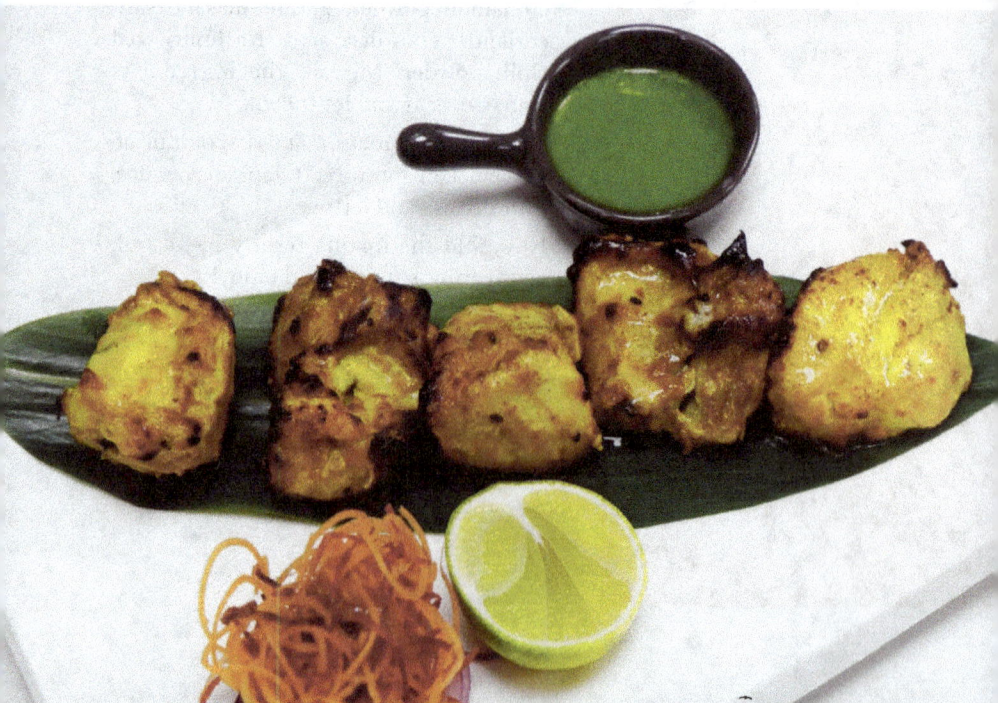

INGREDIENTS:

- For marination:
- 250 grams Fish
- 1/2 tsp red chilli powder 1/2 tsp coriander powder 1/4 tsp turmeric powder 1/2 tsp garam Masala
- 1 tsp raw mango powder (amchur)
- 1/2 tsp mustard oil
- 1 chopped green chilli
- 2 tsp chopped coriander leaves
- 2 tsp curd
- 1 tsp lemon juice
- Salt according to your taste
- 1 tsp ginger garlic paste

GARNISH:

- Chopped coriander leaves

DIRECTIONS:

1. To marinate the fish, take a bowl and add mustard oil, chopped coriander, green chillies, ginger garlic paste, and curd.

2. Then add red chilli powder, salt, garam masala, coriander powder, turmeric, raw mango powder, and lemon juice. Mix it well.

3. Add fish into the marinade and coat the fish properly. Keep it in the fridge for 2-3 hours for best results. So that all the marinate reaches the fish properly.

4. Take a non-stick pan and put the fish in the pan without adding oil to it.

5. Cook the fish from one side for approximately 5-6 minutes on a high flame. It will get the chars as you get from the tandoor.

6. Turn the fish and repeat the same process for another side.

7. Take a plate and plate your fish. Add some chopped coriander leaves over the fish to garnish it. Also, keep some onions, tomatoes and half lemon on the plate and enjoy!

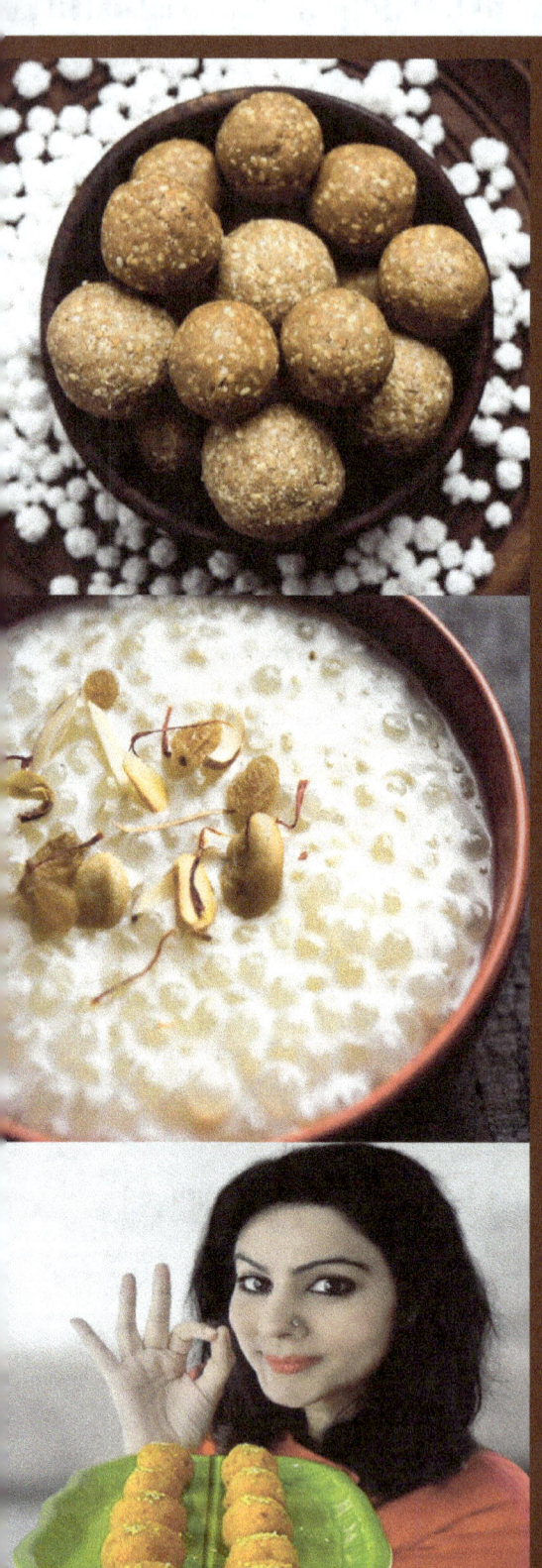

DESSERT

The idea of consuming something sweet during your weight journey seems so impossible. As sugar is considered a food that is known to gain the most of your weight. But, sometimes, in your weight loss journey, you get sugar cravings that you can't resist. And all you think about is sweet food.

We feel that the weight loss journey gets so tedious if you are not allowed to eat your favourite food. That is why we believe you should enjoy your journey! You should devour all the cravings you get on your journey. Be it sweet! Additionally devouring, the dessert is also known to burst all your stress and provide you with immense pleasure. So, to satisfy your sugar craving and fill your life with joy, we have got you your favourite recipes, Laddoo and kheer! These are so delicious that you won't be able to resist. And why should you ignore these? Because these contain so few calories that you can relish them without gaining any weight. These are weight loss dessert recipes!

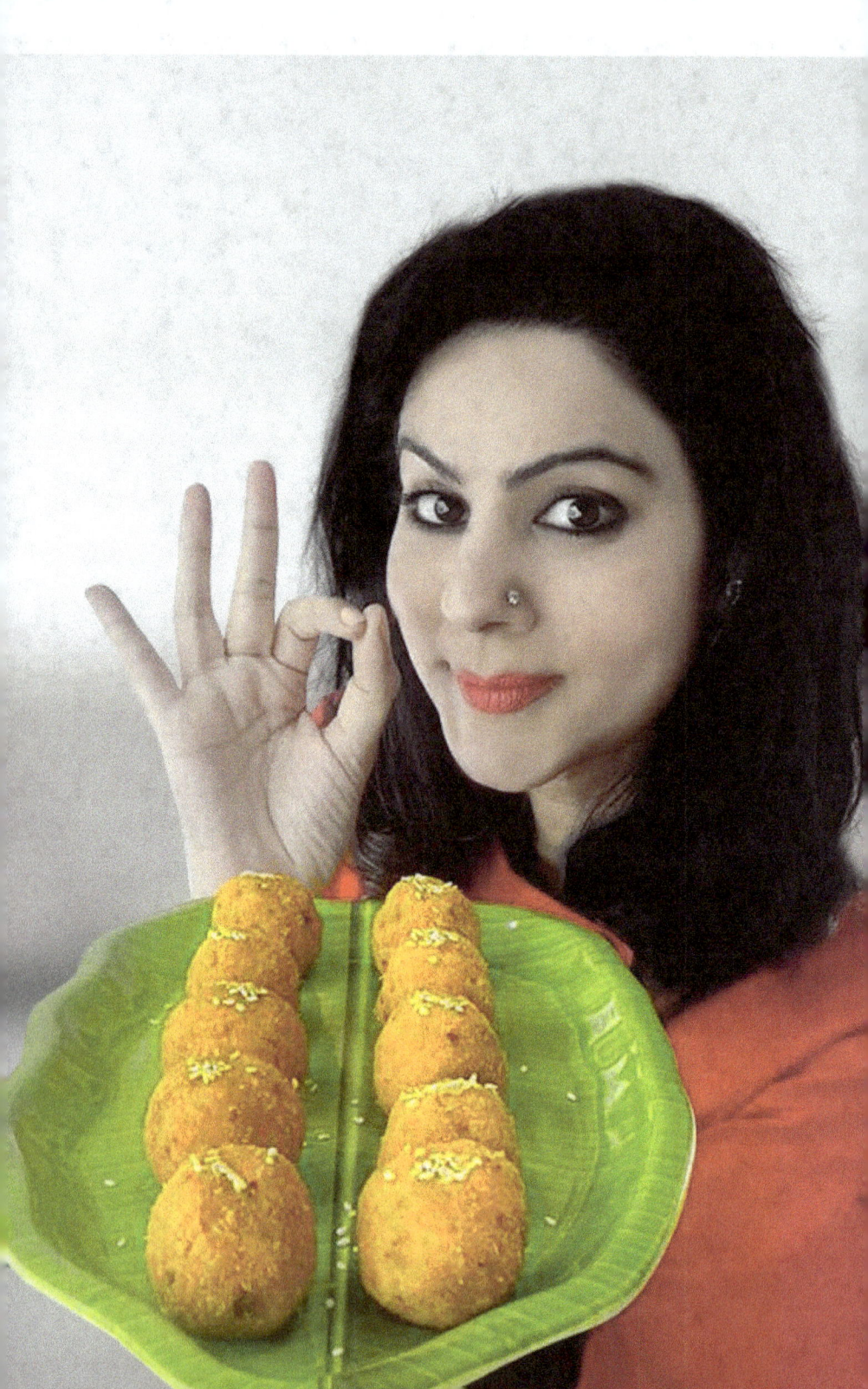

CARROT LADDOO

Ever heard of healthy laddoos? Then, it's the perfect recipe for you! Try our most amazing and healthy carrot laddoo recipe. We guarantee you'll love it! Lose weight with taste as it's only 53 calories per laddoo.

INGREDIENTS:

- 100 grams grated carrot
- 100 grams grated coconut
- 30 grams deseeded dates
- 5 grams cinnamon powder

DIRECTIONS:

1. In a blender add grated carrot, coconut, dates, and cinnamon powder. Blend the ingredients well.
2. Transfer the mixture into a bowl.
3. Use your hands and give this mixture a ball shape. Only take 1 tbsp mixture each to make the laddoo.
4. Garnish the laddoos with sesame seeds and enjoy!

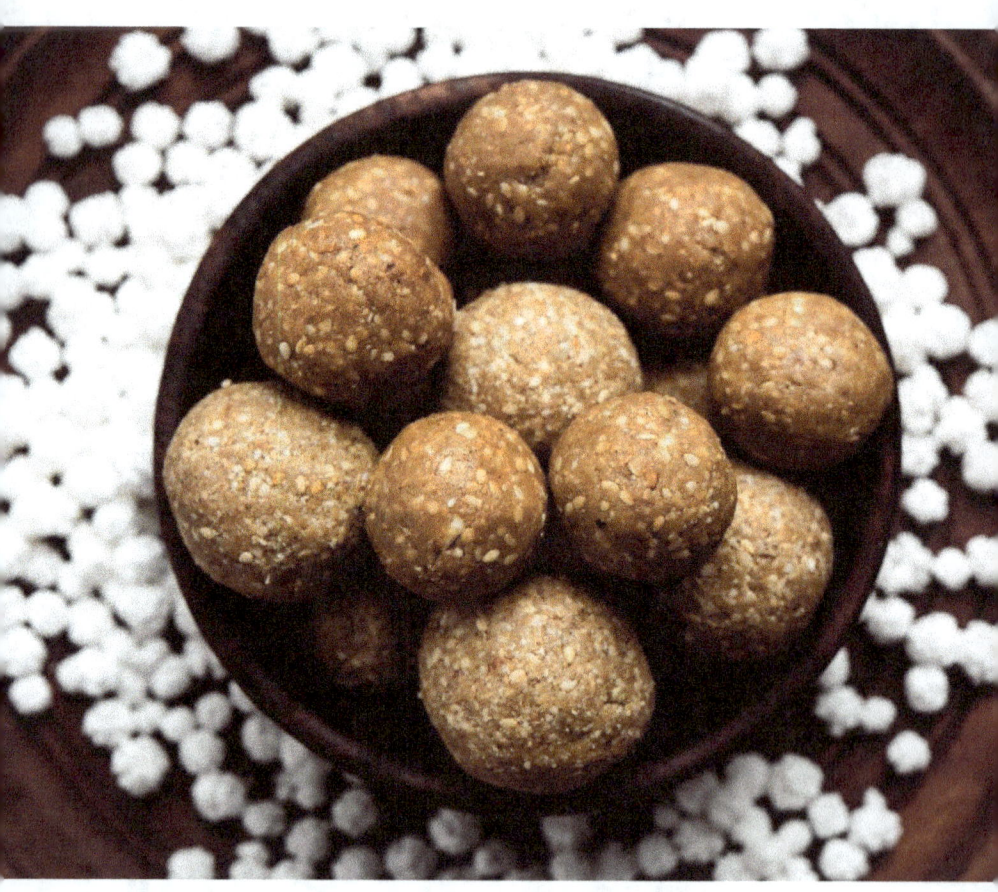

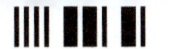 

DATES & ALMOND LADDOO

Craving for some laddoo? Try this mouth-watering laddoo recipe and get a chance to relish your favourite laddoo without any stress of being fat! It's only 66 calories per laddoo! You can easily devour these in your journey.

INGREDIENTS:

- Approximately 20-25 pieces of almonds (soaked and peeled)
- 10-15 pieces of walnuts
- 7-8 pieces pitted dates
- 1 tsp cinnamon powder
- 1 tbsp roasted flaxseeds

DIRECTIONS:

1. In a blender, add almonds, walnut, dates, cinnamon powder, and roasted flaxseeds. Blend it until coarsely ground.

2. Transfer the mixture into a bowl. Using a tsp take the mixture and give it a ball shape. Don't take more than a tsp.

3. Make the laddoos and put them on a plate and, voilà, laddoos are ready, enjoy!

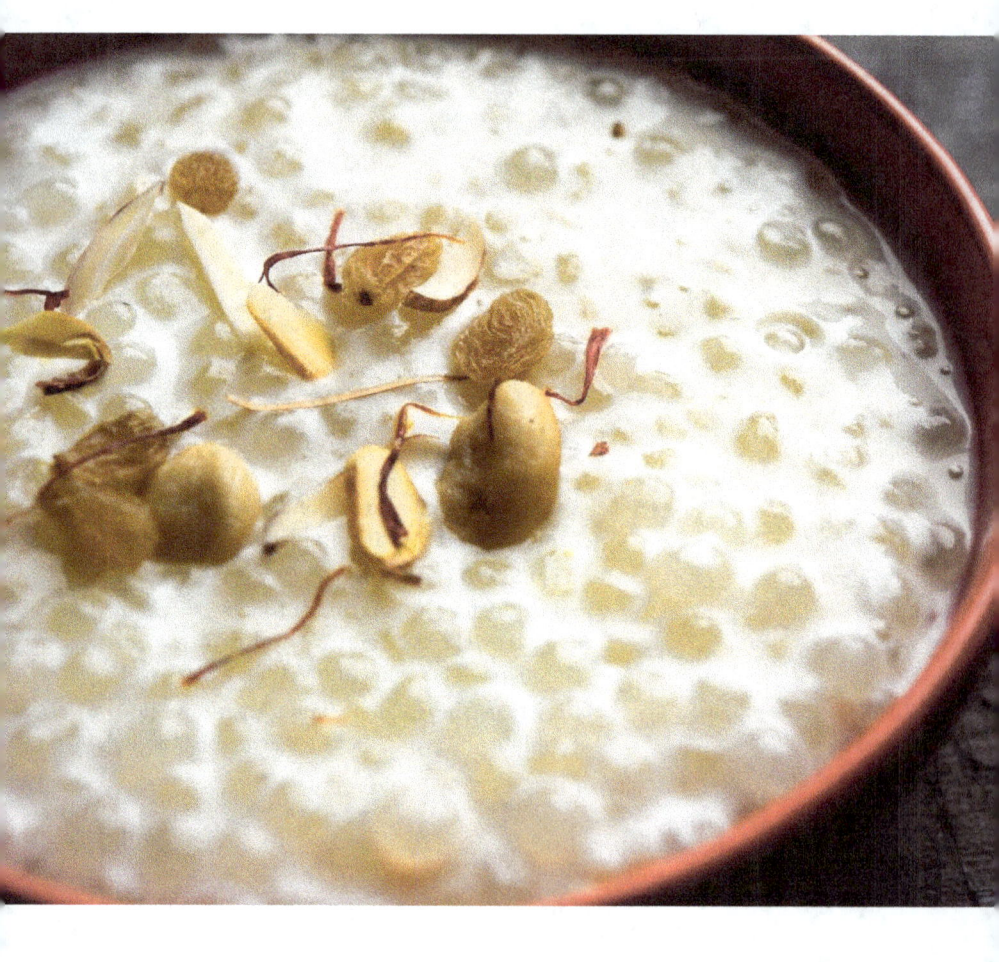

KHEER

Who says you cannot devour sweets in your weight loss journey? Well, with this 16 calories kheer recipe you can! You can even enjoy this during Navratri. It's made with sabudana rice and is very healthy!

INGREDIENTS:

- 100 ml low-fat milk
- 1 tbsp overnight soaked sabudana
- 1/2 glass water
- 1 tsp jaggery powder (organic)
- A pinch of saffron
- 1 tsp soaked and chopped walnut
- 1 tsp soaked, peeled and chopped almond
- 1 tsp soaked and chopped pistachio
- A pinch of cardamom powder

DIRECTIONS:

1. In a saucepan, add 100 ml of low-fat milk to it. Next, add soaked sabudana and approximately 1/2 glass of water.

2. Now, add 1 tsp of jaggery powder. Cover it with a lid and cook until the milk starts to get thick.

3. Next, add a pinch of saffron and let it boil. Cook until it reaches your desired consistency on a low flame.

4. Now, add soaked walnut, soaked almond, and soaked pistachio. Let it boil for a few minutes.

5. Next, add a pinch of cardamom powder. Mix it well.

6. Transfer the kheer into a bowl, and you can have it hot or cold. Enjoy!

Hungry For More?

For more healthy recipes that you can devour in your weight loss journey without any stress of gaining weight, check out my social media pages! I post nutritious recipes there every day!

🌐 https://www.natashamohan.com/

▶ WeightLossWithNatashaMohan

▶ DietRecipesByNatashaMohan

▶ FoodVsHealthHindiTV

f DietitianNatashaMohan

📷 dt.natashamohan

I hope you relish these recipes and make the most out of them! Thank you!

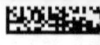